The Jossey-Bass Health Series brings together the most current information and ideas in health care from the leaders in the field. Titles from the Jossey-Bass Health Series include these essential health care resources:

Raising Standards in American Health Care

Raising Standards in American Health Care

Best People, Best Practices, Best Results

V. Clayton Sherman

Jossey-Bass Publishers • San Francisco

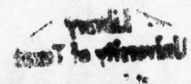

Jossey-Bass books and products are available through most bookstores. To contact Jossey-Bass directly, call (888) 378-2537, fax to (800) 605-2665, or visit our website at www.josseybass.com.

Substantial discounts on bulk quantities of Jossey-Bass books are available to corporations, professional associations, and other organizations. For details and discount information, contact the special sales department at Jossey-Bass.

 Manufactured in the United States of America on Lyons Falls Turin Book. This paper is acid-free and 100 percent totally chlorine-free.

Library of Congress Cataloging-in-Publication Data
Sherman, V. Clayton.
 Raising standards in American health care : best people, best practices, best results / V. Clayton Sherman.
  p.   cm.
Includes bibliographical references and index.
ISBN 0-7879-4621-4 (hardcover : alk. paper)
1. Medical care — Standards — United States. 2. Social medicine — Standards — United States.   I. Title.
RA395.A3S483   1999
362.1′02′1873 — dc21

                                                        98-53278
                                                        CIP

FIRST EDITION
HB Printing   10 9 8 7 6 5 4 3 2 1

Contents

Preface

I entered consulting in 1978 after a dozen years working in corporate America. What I experienced was nothing less than culture shock as I encountered an approach to management that was woefully behind the revolution that was then occurring in business and industry. Driven by merciless competition from Japan and Europe, American management had forsaken disproved management concepts and was retooling their industries. This was the era of the Chrysler rescue and the Harley Davidson resurgence. Business was learning the painful lesson that unless you change how you manage, you had better update your resume. That learning paid off as American business took strong center stage in the 1990s as an evolved management system produced magnificent results.

Where was health care during that era? As a presenter I couldn't talk about "profit" or "customer" in the early 1980s without having audiences react in shock. Health care as an industry was in a time warp, notably behind the advance of the management profession and seemingly oblivious to its direction. Much has greatly changed, and health care management has moved a long way past the stagnation caused by the old cost-reimbursement model that held up normal industry evolution. At this moment, we're still catching up to the state of the management art—gaining rapidly but not yet there.

Americans love the direction health care is moving—new technology, new services, new solutions. What they hate is a cost picture caused by system inefficiencies that bankrupts recipients and payers. These inefficiencies result either from services performed at too low a level (a standards problem) or by using approaches that have not been standardized on best practices. On the quality front, health care has become the scandal of the week in the media. Removal of wrong limbs, medication poisonings, and malpractice cases provide plentiful grist for the news mill. These terrible results come despite the best management efforts, thus frustrating providers and frightening Customers. Something is *systemically* wrong with health care, not just in its work processes but in how it is managed.

What the Book Is About

This is a book about changing the American health care system by changing the *standards* that govern it. It presents what used to be defined as a quality issue but is now a critical management problem—standards are too low, often inappropriate, and sometimes nonexistent. Ultimately, inadequate standards, a lack of measures to judge appropriate performance, and ill-defined work procedures combine to create horrible, out-of-control consequences for patients and out-of-control performance for organizations. From a management perspective, these outcomes are unacceptable.

This is also a book about *standardization*—about removing variations in equipment, procedures, professional practice, and organizational performances. Standardization to best practices is the cure—standardization of defined clinical protocols, in management and nonclinical functions, between operating units, even standardization around the Golden Rule, because only well-treated people can treat Customers well. Why standardization across the board? Because standardization, and only standardization, can produce the low-cost, high-quality service outcomes that Customers demand and have every right to expect.

Where does one start to write a book on the need to change the American health care system? The subject is so broad, complex, and diverse that any approach must quickly concentrate on some workable propositions. The frame of reference I chose for the book is a management perspective on internal organization operations. The focus is primarily on how to make provider organizations into clean, lean machines—that is, highly efficient, highly effective deliverers of one of the most needed products in America. My aim is to provide concepts and tools to leaders in the field. The book is based on important findings in management research, but its focus is on the application of this knowledge by top executives and departmental managers. It provides a set of ideas and techniques to help leaders change the organization and radically improve its ability to get results. It's all about making the shop run right.

Many health professions are struggling to define clinical practice protocols. I support this work in the arguments I make for raising standards, standards that are defined by best practices in all aspects of health care. Physicians, nurses, radiology and laboratory technicians, and all other professionals who have been actively engaged in defining standards and wrestling with standardization issues will find the management approach I am recommending compatible and supportive. What is still missing is an organization- and industrywide awareness that this is the critical issue and we must face it together. We need a plan the whole team can rally around.

How do we get an entire industry to upgrade itself? Renewal on an individual hospital basis, each unit having to start from ground zero, is a slow, unwieldy approach to the needs of the industry. It is like having a tailor make a custom suit by hand. Although the quality is great, the result takes a long time and costs a lot to achieve. A better idea would be an off-the-rack product that anyone could wear now and at half the cost. Smaller institutions, particularly, don't have the staff time to do it all themselves or the budget to be able to afford help from high-priced consultants. And to gain some degree of commonality in large systems, it would be helpful if at least core pieces were "plug and play." That realization produced the urge to write this book.

Employers and business coalitions have been driving much of the managed care revolution by contracting with providers who can measure and demonstrate favorable *cost, quality, and customer satisfaction outcomes*. Their tough insistence on numeric targets reflects a mindset that is at the core of all modern management practice—if you don't measure it, you can't manage it. As corporate managements see it, providers have to meet standards in these three areas or they'll find providers who will. Providers can meet that challenge by pursuing standards and the emerging concept of strategic standardization. This book will help bridge to the new management approaches required to compete in the future.

Perspectives and Limitations

In the ancient fable, seven blind men all described an elephant differently based on the part of the anatomy they encountered. The blind man who grabbed the tail thought of the elephant as a rope. The blind man who encountered the leg thought of the animal as a tree. Each had a different perception, somewhat accurate but insufficient. There are a lot of opinions right now about how to manage our health care organizations better. Each is right, in a way, but each suffers from an insufficiency, an inadequacy of approach. This book was designed to put together a range of ideas that, when taken together, may serve to provide a more workable road map for producing dramatically better organizational performance.

Although I have been schooled in various management orientations (total quality management [TQM], management by objective [MBO], human resources, finance, operations analysis, strategic planning, organization development), I don't believe any of these orientations have a lock on the truth. Effective organizations follow the management dictate of doing what works. They are eclectic and reject the narrow mindset of any one school of thought. The reader who is a continuous improvement devotee will be pleased with many of my comments but infuriated at my many departures from that doctrine. In like fashion, some elements of what I propose will seem familiar and comfortable to every reader, no matter what their orientation to management, and some will sound strange at first. In twenty years of working in over 700 client hospitals and health systems and in another 300 organizations in business and industry, I have learned to focus solely on the question of what works rather than pledging allegiance to a narrow orthodoxy.

My consulting experience has been mostly with individual profit and nonprofit general hospitals. In recent years an increasing percentage of my practice has been in working with health care systems as they have evolved. Many of the examples in this book come from that background. These examples demonstrate the complexity of the old core hospital business, particularly the difficult challenges of doing organization change work there, and the linkage for shared services it provides to other nonhospital-based services. Although some readers will wish for more examples from home health, nursing homes, health maintenance organizations (HMOs), public and military hospitals, and group medical practice, the same principles of standardization apply. Managers in all aspects of health care will have little difficulty in understanding the message or applying it.

In a way, the new approach to management is uniquely American. Running deep in our "can do" culture is a belief that we can make things better by using a lot of energy and a little common sense. Ours is an activist management style known as *effectiveness*—both brainy and gutsy. Effectiveness is the acid test: Does it work? Does it make a difference? In health care today those questions must be asked. The answers will often show that the time to replace the ineffective approaches that haven't been working has come.

Will these ideas work in other countries? I don't know. Maybe there's something universal about them that would find success anywhere. What I do know is that these ideas have been tested here, they work here, and they succeed rapidly when aggressively implemented. It is a doable American dream: happy customers, high quality, low cost, and turned-on staff. The message of this book is that if we manage differently, if we raise standards in everything we do, we can produce a very big difference in how our health care organizations perform. The promise of this book is that if we rethink our assumptions and then remake our organizations, the dream can come true.

Corporate Benchmarks

Throughout the book I refer to benchmark management practices in the corporate world. I have been consistently encouraged by the larger management community to make the arguments found herein and not to pull any punches in making them. It is clearly the wish of the management community to see a far higher level of management performance in health care. Until health care management performs at higher levels, the quality and cost problems that now beset the industry will not improve sufficiently. In this contest, winning is defined by results, not by how hard we tried or how much we cared.

I refer particularly to three companies that offer clear examples of what strategic standardization can mean if practiced in health care organizations: McDonald's, Wal-Mart, and Southwest Airlines.

I chose them because they are well known to most readers, and this familiarity allows us to critique whether these management concepts should apply to hospitals. All of these organizations

- Operate in highly competitive industries where systems are fully advanced
- Are rated number one in their respective industries
- Have performed at high levels for many years, showing a consistency of performance through variations in market and economic cycles

None of these corporations is perfect. But they've earned the notable distinction of being widely accepted by the marketplace and are dominant against their competitors. They have achieved their strategic objectives of quality, cost, and service through the effective utilization of their people. Their strategy, known as Operational Excellence, is the one that health care organizations must now implement.

When considering how to develop a new hospital organization model, comparing the new model against that of organizations pursuing a similar market strategy is important. I chose these examples because they represent a more fully developed picture of the intensity and extensiveness that hospitals must emulate. Best practices and benchmarks have to be taken where you find them.

Work-Out Sessions

At the end of each chapter I've included a number of suggested questions for discussion. Their value is in helping readers apply the ideas of that chapter. These questions can be asked by a project team assigned to look at the elements of standardization, or by an individual manager analyzing what is needed in her department. Managers at a department head meeting might gather in several groups, each to discuss and report on one of the questions. The questions, and the book, are to be used as a springboard to action.

Language

I capitalize the words Customer and Associate (employee) wherever they appear. Although this practice may flout the conventions of grammar, keeping the importance of these two central groups in clear focus is simply good management, one that many health care organizations are now following. Think of it this way: Capitalizing these two words is a no-cost way to communicate something very valuable to these audiences—and to keep our own thinking straight.

The pronouns *he* and *she* are inclusive of both sexes and are not meant to suggest limits. At this point in health care, we need all the help we can get. It's not a matter of equal opportunity as much as it is a matter of equal responsibility. Everyone is needed, everyone must respond. No one should be left out, no one should be left behind.

Supplemental Texts

Effective leaders define themselves primarily as *professionals in management,* and only secondarily as *health care* managers. They take the broader view of their profession and are inclusive in their conceptual base about how to pursue solutions. For hundreds of practical examples that are specific to health care and extend the concepts of this book, refer to *Total Customer Satisfaction* (1998) by Stephanie Sherman and published by Jossey-Bass, part of a planned series, *Strategies for Health Care Excellence.* More volumes are under development that will address issues of people, quality, and cost. The present book can be thought of as the umbrella work over the entire series, laying out broad issues that the other books then examine in detail. Together with this book, these volumes will represent the completion of a body of work that we began with our 1993 offering, *Creating the New American Hospital.* It was our intention that management teams work their way through the series, implementing as they go, using each book as a "change module."

The Book's Contents

The book looks first at what the market demands and needs, and then at the kind of organizational structure, goals, and processes that can deliver the needed results. The book then discusses the next link in the chain: installing the work procedures and protocols that represent best practices, everywhere, in all departments. Finally, the book looks at how to deal with impediments to change that keep all this wonderful stuff from happening.

Part One: The Need to Move to Higher Ground

The book begins by focusing on the two essential foundation stones necessary to both raise health care's standards and to improve its business performance. Chapter One, "The Rebirth of Health Care Management," makes the argument that the revolution in how leaders manage health care must be completed. A defined system of managing must be brought to bear on the problem of management variance. Organizational performance will not improve until managerial performance improves. The man in the mirror is where change begins. Our management teams will find in this chapter some of the new techniques and tools they need to succeed. Chapter Two, "The Strategy-Standards Equation," examines the first law of management: Obey the market. Here you'll find three exciting tools: a simple-to-communicate strategy called Operational Excellence, the balanced scorecard, and stretch goals. Together they function remarkably well in giving everybody a clear picture of where we're headed. Part One says, If it is to be, it's up to me—and here's the map that will get us to the promised land.

Part Two: Redefining American Health Care Standards

The cost and quality problems of the industry result primarily from pursuing or tolerating standards that are too low. Chapter Three, "Winning with Strategic Standardization," shows how a new approach being used in business and industry—aggressively raising standards—produces competitive advantage and reliably meets market demands for better outcomes. In Chapter Four, "Existing Standards Are Not Enough," we will look at why current standards are unacceptable and will seek standards that are higher than those of accrediting agencies. Meeting these standards will produce phenomenal success.

Part Three: Commonsense Solutions for Uncommon Performance

Here will be found the commonsense solutions needed to move from current to higher levels of performance. Much of this is the nitty-gritty all managers look for, the practical approaches to making change. Chapter Five, "Moving to McDonaldland," an extended case study, compares standardization in one of the world's most successful organizations with that in health care organizations and points to what the latter must now do. One example is the incredibly different picture of how suppliers are utilized.

Chapter Six, "Creating a New American Hospital," describes an organizational model that is capable of transitioning the organization to higher levels and delivering on the promise of higher standards. It is the "horse to ride" in terms of a new delivery vehicle for services and incorporates the new management methods described in Chapter One.

Chapter Seven, "Competing on Knowledge," examines the new currency of intellectual capital. Most important, it demonstrates how this truer measure of business worth can be multiplied and used to massive advantage. One clear picture that emerges is that twenty-first century health care organizations will win based primarily on their ability to do best thinking.

Best thinking comes only from best people. Chapter Eight, "First Feed the Troops," lays out what must be done to form a new employment contract of trust with Associates. The trust damaged by layoffs and less than best human management practices is sizable and must be repaired. At the same time, new approaches must be created to realigning jobs and staffing. First, *best people*, then *best practices*. Finally, *best results*.

Chapter Nine, "Best Practices Make Perfect," is a chapter on tools for best practices and benchmarking. The task here is to copy best practices when you can find them, invent them when you can't. The demanding aspect of this part of the equation is that all practices, in all areas of the organization, must be replaced with best practices. A complete rebuilding job is required—no less. There's a lot of work to do.

Part Four: Change Managing the Standardization Process

The final part of the book is all about getting from point A to point B: how to move your organization, or your people, or your suppliers, from today's to tomorrow's performance. The process of standardization begins by figuring out a success path. Chapter Ten, "Defeating the Limits of Change," looks at the factors for which change masters must make allowances, and how they can work through the resistance barriers. Chapter Eleven, "Transforming Health Care Organizations," is a step-by-step application of the actual renewal plan that is useful for single-facility or multi-unit systems transformations.

Who the Book Is For

I wrote this book for people in health care management, wherever they are working. I doubt there's a tougher job in management right now. I thought about how the book might help people in provider organizations and those who serve them, particularly

- Hospital boards and top management
- System organization leaders and those working on integration problems
- Long-term care, home health care, and psychiatric facilities
- Department leaders and supervisors
- Managers of clinics and ambulatory care centers
- Physicians and group practice managers
- Suppliers of all kinds

But the book also has value for the people who have to bear the economic burden, who are vitally concerned about the performance of their contracting providers and the reactions of served Customers:

- Managers in managed care organizations and HMOs
- Employers and business coalitions
- Insurance companies and health plans

A third group consists of those who primarily focus on standards, quality, and education issues:

- Faculty in graduate programs who are creating the new leadership
- Accrediting and licensing organization leaders
- Professional associations
- New knowledge specialists in consulting, organization development, quality, reengineering, and customer satisfaction
- Government regulators at all levels

This book is a reflection of the commitment already made, and the direction already taken, by the men and women of American health care who are moving us to higher ground. Some of the concepts or wording may be new, but the elements will feel immediately at home in the enhanced organizations we're creating. Raising standards in American health care is our calling, our opportunity, and our privilege. It is time to rise and shine.

Acknowledgments

Special thanks to friends, family, faculty, mentors, and so many clients who had the courage to try this stuff out, and whose successes taught me so much. Thanks to critics who said it couldn't be done—it was fun proving them wrong. Thanks to Andy Pasternack at Jossey-Bass, who understood the need for this book and its supplemental series, and acted as patient godfather. Thanks to the infants, the ill and dying, the oldsters who have no voice—I tried to speak for you all. Thanks America for always holding high the lamp and for being the Land of the Second Chance. Thanks Dad. Thanks Mom. I'm still trying.

April 1999

V. CLAYTON SHERMAN
Inverness, Illinois

For Nola

*In memory of a beloved sister, whose high standards
challenged others, and whose early departure has moved us
to redouble our efforts.*

For Adam, Andrew, Ben, Emily, J. B., and Jon

*In hope that our children will have better, healthier lives,
and that they will be better served by a healthier
American health care system.*

But most of all, for Steffie

*Whose strength of mind is more than I can keep up with,
and whose strength of heart is more than I deserve.*

The Author

V. Clayton Sherman is chairman of Management House, Inc. in Inverness, Illinois. Management House provides management development, organizational renewal, and human resource services to a wide range of health care organizations, Fortune 500 companies, and associations. Clay holds an MBA and doctorate in management education from Western Michigan University, and did postdoctoral work at Harvard University's Graduate School of Business Administration in the area of managing organizational effectiveness. Clay has also studied under Dr. W. Edwards Deming in London. He is the author of seven management books, including *Creating the New American Hospital,* which has helped many hospitals dramatically improve organizational performance. Using his management approaches, his clients have won Top 100 status, received the American Hospital Association's Great Comebacks Award, the Society for Human Resources Management's Innovative Practices Award, the Global Best Practices Award for Customer Service, 3-M's Innovations in Health Care, and have achieved Customer satisfaction ratings for best in nation. He is in great demand as one of America's best speakers, and is frequently quoted as an expert on management by radio, television, and print media.

Prologue

In 1841, a young Hungarian physician Ignaz Semmelweiss (1818–1865) was hired to run a maternity unit in a Vienna training hospital used mainly by the poor. There were two birthing wards, one run by midwives and the other by doctors. Semmelweiss noted that death rates among mothers in the doctors' ward were much higher than those in the midwives' ward; most of the women died from an infection called childbed fever. When he suggested that doctors might be contributing to this, he was fired.

Once background politics played themselves out, Semmelweiss was rehired. After witnessing a friend die subsequent to cutting himself during an autopsy of a patient who had died of childbed fever, Semmelweiss reasoned that an "invisible agent" was being carried from the autopsy room and infecting mothers during birthing. He instituted sanitary measures, requiring all doctors to wash their hands and change from blood-soaked lab coats after autopsies.

And the result? His patients lived. Death rates dropped by two-thirds. Babies grew up, heard their mothers sing songs, learned to ride horses, were counseled by fathers, went off to school, had families of their own—thanks to Dr. Semmelweiss.

Physicians still objected to Semmelweiss's new procedures, however, and he was again fired. He was expelled from the medical society; notices ridiculing him appeared in the press. He and his family became social outcasts. Driven from one job to another, he nonetheless instituted the same cleanliness standards at each job and hospital, which resulted in the same decline in deaths and the same angry reaction from fellow physicians. To the very end of his short life he fought for a simple change, and was castigated for it. He paid a terrific price for his simple idea. But his patients lived.

Thirty years later, Dr. Joseph Lister was knighted for demonstrating independently the value of handwashing and for pioneering antiseptics. Lister gave full credit to Semmelweiss, saying that surgery could not have advanced without his insight.

Standards come with a price. Today the price is work, a lot of it. Semmelweiss paid the price that was called for in his day. He became a hero.

Now it's your turn.

Raising Standards in American Health Care

Part One

The Need to Move to Higher Ground

The heights by great men reached and kept
Were not attained by sudden flight,
But they, while their companions slept,
Were toiling upward in the night.
—HENRY WADSWORTH LONGFELLOW

If there is a universal characteristic of effective leaders, it is that they are never satisfied with things as they are. They want to change things because it is part of acting out their own needs for achievement, for making a difference. In a sense, they are users of their organizations. They use them to contribute, to do good, to show that it mattered that they were here. These people, and you are among them, are about to revolutionize American health care. The opportunity is all about standards and how to take health care to a whole new level. The test of these leaders will be whether they can make health care operationally excellent.

Chapter One

The Rebirth of Health Care Management

Pronouncing our intentions, and actually acting on them, are two entirely different matters. It's like the general who issued a rousing battle cry: "Onward to victory!" Half an hour later, an urgent message reached him from an officer in the field: "Need further instructions. Victory not on our maps."

With this chapter we begin an exciting journey. We examine what management has to do to create new health care delivery systems that perform at higher levels than anything we've seen yet. We'll also look at the wrecks along the way—the failed approaches in management that must now be abandoned, for health care's problems stem primarily from a set of management assumptions that are no longer useful. We will look at a new set of understandings that can revitalize existing organizations and provide an environment in which new health care delivery elements can flourish. We begin with this most basic understanding: The work of remaking organizations begins with leaders that are so ethically accountable, so committed, that they are willing to remake their approach to managing. *Raising standards finds its genesis in better management performance.*

Management's New Opportunity

The Emperor Shi Huangdi, the first leader to unify the Chinese empire, built the Great Wall in the third century B.C. by linking earlier walls of states along the northern frontier with Mongolia as a means to thwart invasion. It is over 1,500 miles long in some of the roughest terrain on earth. Fifteen to forty feet wide and twenty to fifty feet high, the wall was built almost entirely by hand. Towns developed at gates placed in the wall. The wall was maintained for almost 1,800 years by successive rulers. Ironically, the Manchu conquerors of the Ming dynasty in the 1500s found the wall to be no obstacle—the gatekeepers were simply bribed (*Grolier Encyclopedia,* 1998). For every complex system, there are always breach points, and they are most often human, not technological. Chinese leaders needed to rethink their system of defense. Instead of relying on what had worked in the past, they should have reexamined their assumptions.

We have created a Great Health Care System, which, though admirable in many respects, is of such complexity that we fear it as a runaway, a system that no one can be sure is reliably in control. Like the Chinese, we have erected elaborate barriers and safeguards, but these are breached by each medication error, surgical misadventure, or cost overrun. Our means seem to work against our ends. The more we try to create and control a stable state, the more unstable things become. Our health care system's errors are caused partly by a lack of technology or by poorly designed work processes, but largely its failings are human, caused primarily by an absence of applied disciplines of management. Those who designed the Great Health Care System, and those who are keepers of its gates, must rethink the system, for its problems are many. In this chapter we examine the role of management in health care's current crisis, both because the leaders are accountable and because they now have a historic opportunity to alter health care delivery for the better.

Today we stand at the gateway of what may well prove to be the most remarkable generation of progress in health care history. Within the lifetime of many current health care leaders, the cures for many of humankind's most feared illnesses may be achieved. Given the successes of health care research and innovation, it is no longer impossible to envision that the plague of AIDS will be gone, cancer will no longer exact its heavy toll of fear and pain, or that heart disease, birth defects, and many problems of the aging will be eradicated. If we can get at the core issues of *strategic standardization,* we will be able to solve the problem of decreased resources and achieve the expansion of care for those without coverage. We will finish the work of system building, accelerate the capabilities we already have to do far more, and exploit opportunities of which we have only now begun to dream. Far from a utopian wish, the speed of medical progress through scientific research, technology's skyrocketing gains, and the will of health care professionals everywhere all make these doable goals if we will do the job of raising standards and implementing best practices in all aspects of operations.

For present-day leaders to realize that all these remarkable breakthroughs are just over the horizon is critically important. Yet the industry suffers from a management system that is inadequate for birthing and cradling twenty-first century health care. It is a management system that needs not just upgrading but replacement. And it is this generation of leaders who will have to transform that system—a challenge that is both a blessing and a curse. It is a curse in the sense that this will take a lot of work with little time, and it is a blessing in that in rising to the challenge, these leaders will be heroes who improve the lives of us all.

Failure analysis is an engineering concept that holds that study of failed designs often yields new knowledge that can improve products and prevent failure in the future. When the Federal Aviation Administration (FAA) examines a crash site, it is performing a type of failure analysis. It's not fun poking in the ashes of yesterday's problems, but if we're going to have a better future, it is necessary work. Those who lead our health care organizations today are committed to making whatever alterations will improve future success. What, then, are the causes for the current failings that we see in our systems of care? How can we design in elements that will improve our individual and organizational performance? Ultimately, the horrors of system-injured patients, or dismal business results, stem from management failure. Can we become comfortable with the idea that saying our management approach needs improvement is not to say that health care managers are failures? As David Packard said, "If you can't make a mistake, you can't make anything." It's OK that mistakes happen; what is not OK is to fail to find out why and to keep letting them happen. Because the failure of a management approach leads to organizational failure, we must understand the causes underlying both halves of the problem.

The Crisis in Health Care Organizations

To understand why organizations fail, we need to understand why organizations succeed. In the early 1980s it was demonstrated that successful organizations shared a common profile of winning practices that, taken together, allowed these companies to dominate. The challenge for organizations was to create peak performance, a notion initially popularized by *In Search of Excellence* by Peters and Waterman (1997). In many cases devising ways to operate at peak performance entailed plain common sense, what Tom Peters and Bob Waterman called, "a blinding flash of the obvious." Factors such as being close to the Customer, utilizing people at full capacity, pushing the limits of innovation, sticking with core businesses, and streamlining work systems all contributed important parts of the puzzle. But what really made the difference in these organizations was their extremism in focusing on these factors, and their spirited human cultures that provided spark and sizzle.

We have also learned there is a profile of failure, just as there is one of winning. *All organizations can fail, and all organizations can improve.* And health care organizations badly need improvement. Organizational failure, like success, occurs for predictable reasons. Understanding this profile can be a positive way to begin to understand why so many health care organizations are struggling and what leadership must change to win. Management's task will be to remove elements of failure and introduce success factors.

Why do organizations fail? They usually fail for one or more of the following seven reasons, all widely found in America's health care industry and all controllable by management. Organizations that do not rush to control these variables are skirting with organizational death. Executives must respond with urgency to these warning signs.

Quality Is "Out of Control"

Extrapolations from the benchmark study conducted by Harvard University for the state of New York to the national population suggest that 1.3 million people are injured annually in hospitals, 100,000 of whom will die. What makes this situation doubly painful is the finding that 335,000 of these injuries are due to negligence, and that of this subgroup, 80,000 will die. These estimates are extrapolations based on the Harvard Medical Practice Study of 37,000 patients discharged from New York hospitals in 1984, in an effort to determine rates of injury caused by medical treatment in hospitals: 3.7 percent of patients suffered injuries due to medical treatment, 28 percent of which were due to negligence. The study concluded that most adverse events were preventable, particularly those due to error or negligence (Brennan, Leape, Laird, and others, 1991; Leape, Brennan, Laird, and others, 1991). More recent studies are coming in with higher estimates. Three studies published in the *Journal of the American Medical Association* indicate that as many as 140,000 people may be dying from adverse drug reactions alone, that 50 percent of these are preventable, and that 75 percent of the preventable half could have been caught by computerized systems, which hospitals have been slow to install ("Drug Prescribing Errors Studied," 1997). At the 1996 "Examining Errors in Health Care" conference sponsored by the American Medical Association (AMA), the Joint Commission on Accreditation of Healthcare Organizations (JCAHO), and others, it was reported that 180,000 Americans die from care received in hospitals, and that another 1.1 million are injured (Shinkman, 1996a).

Although estimates vary, they're all huge and indicate a system not yet adequately managed. That so many should be injured or killed by their hospital encounter gives the hospital industry one of the highest error rates of any industry in the United States. The public's growing disenchantment is evidenced by media exposés and court actions.

To some degree the industry has been in a state of denial about this quality problem. In the famous 1995 Dana-Farber incident in which Betsy Lehman, health columnist for the *Boston Globe*, died as a result of medication error, management took aggressive action to confront the problem. Said James Conway, COO of Dana-Farber, "We should stop saying errors are rare and admit they're everywhere." He also suggests that those who self-report should be thanked, not blamed, and that changing systems and work processes with specific error reduction goals is better than dealing with these problems on a per incident basis. Proper management is forthright, and creates an open culture in which problem solving becomes the order of the day. Failure in health care is a horrible error, but far more horrible is not performing failure analysis. By learning better, we can manage better.

But the denial problem goes on. Least helpful are the claims still heard that "American health care is the best in the world." This jingoistic chauvinism varnishes over the too real problems of medication errors, surgical misadventures, and laboratory fiascos. The public isn't fooled by this industry self-deception. The 1995 Florida case in which a patient's foot was amputated in error (they were supposed to amputate the other one) may have been no different from many others of its kind, but it received particular notoriety. Such cases eliminate any pretense that the layman is unable to understand medical complexity: The average citizen concludes that the health care system simply can't tell the left foot from the right.

Although it can rightfully be claimed that care in the United States, on average, is good, that comparison fails to look at the range of variability. At one end of the spectrum, the U.S. health care industry delivers world-class care, literally as good as that done anywhere. But at the other end, the industry kills 100,000 people and injures twelve times as many, or it provides no care at all to isolated populations. It is that negative deviation from the average that's the problem. The challenge is clear: Reduce the variance at the low end of performance, and continue to raise performance levels at the high end.

A brief technical interpretation. In quality management terms, performance is said to be "out of control" when variance from the mean is too great. Assuming that some mistakes are likely to happen, at what point do we conclude that they are occurring at above the normal rate? For the sake of illustration, the number of times that people tend to make mistakes—their expected error rate (EER)—is six times per thousand. Six per thousand is the number of times one might expect to misdial the telephone, make a wrong turn when driving a known route, or miscount medication. The error rate of American hospitals is 38 per thousand admissions. Is that just a little high, or are we witnessing a situation that is "out of control"? A simplified formula for determining whether we are within a statistically acceptable range is to calculate the upper and lower control limits. Using an EER of 6 as the mean, the formula would be

$$UCL/LCL = X \pm 3\sqrt{X} = 6 \pm 3\sqrt{6} = 0 \text{ to } 13.35 \text{ errors }/1000$$

Assuming that EER is a good standard of comparison, we can state with 99 percent certainty that the system is "out of control." In such circumstances, action must be taken by management to change the system. In actual practice, comparing one hospital's errors against others in its peer group represents a better standard. But consider this, if nearly all hospitals are underperforming, are peer group standards worth pursuing?

Consider the quality problem through analogy. For the airline industry to kill 100,000 people a year would require crashing 285 fully loaded Boeing 747s annually, about six per week. We saw how much agony and investigation went into determining the cause of the TWA 800 crash off Long Island in 1996. It's reasonable to assume the FAA would ground the entire airline industry if it had the same kill rate as America's hospitals. It's been suggested that the reason the industry doesn't draw the same amount of investigative fury is because the 100,000 die one at a time. Obfuscation surrounds these incidents—the victim was "too old," the reason "natural causes," there were "complications" following surgery, or "contributive factors" in a complex biological system.

Make no mistake, this is not muckraking nor is it meant as a diatribe against tremendously dedicated caregivers. It can be argued that making a quality automobile, or flying passengers in intercontinental jets, is an easier job than mastering the greater complexity of health care. But defending errors in the name of their management difficulty is certainly counterproductive. It is a true quandary, for we are dealing with problems that are tremendously complex, over which we often have insufficient knowledge or control. For the most part in health care, people struggle, often heroically, to deliver the premier products of a life saved or condition healed. But it would be criminal to hide instances in which inability to achieve success was caused by a lousy work system, incompetent practitioners, or too-low standards. How good do you think our system is—world-class or error ridden? In your mind, you just set a standard. One thing we can say with certainty about current quality levels: Just as today's patient or practitioner would not accept the quality standards of twenty years ago, no one in the early twenty-first century will accept the standards of today. *We have a quality problem and it must be resolved.*

Prescription. A starting point might be to find out why TQM and other quality initiatives failed in 80 percent of health care applications. Motorola required that quality be the first agenda item for every meeting in every department for the last fifteen years. How frequently is it acted on in your organization? Where are the quality goals and measures? Are managers who achieve the mark rewarded? Are they removed if they don't?

Rampant Bureaucratic Muck

Walt Bogdanich, Pulitzer Prize winning journalist and author of the health care exposé, *The Great White Lie,* wrote of the hospital industry's "dirty little secrets: waste, greed, incompetence—plus enough bureaucratic arrogance to rival the Kremlin" ("Tale of Health Care Could Induce Nausea," 1991). Although it was the "waste, greed, and incompetence" targets that Bogdanich was most interested in pillorying, it's the "bureaucratic arrogance" problem that may be more truly revealing of industry problems, and more centrally important to finding solutions. We now know that organizations that are *swift and flexible* have proven successful in other industries and will probably carry the day in their competitive wars. Yet what we see in health care is heavier *external bureaucracies* among regulators, payers, and business groups and a heavier *internal bureaucratic load* caused by the emergence of system hierarchies on top of already top-heavy hospital organizational structures. These bureaucracies slow down organizational performance rather than get to the heart of problems swiftly— exactly the wrong response for a situation requiring urgency.

Organizational failure is typically associated with complacency and organizational bloat. In such cultures, management drifts and people either don't work very hard or work hard on work that hardly matters. One sees in many of the new systems a heavy overhead of system executives pasted on top of the old, individual hospital hierarchy. What do these people do? What do they contribute? If operating units are moving more slowly, it's time to rethink.

Prescription. Set up a paperwork reduction task force. Have a team of middle managers review the policy manual for unnecessarily restrictive elements. Cut requisition signatures in half. In cases of severe organizational strangulation, turnaround histories suggest that what's most often needed is a new boss who will provide a good, hard shake-up and a management team prepared to do more than just go to another useless meeting and stick with the status quo. Corporate transformation work has shown that without a serious injection of new thinking at the top, organizational performance is not likely to improve ("A Master Class in Radical Change," 1993).

Out of Touch with Customers

Another problem the industry faces is the highest litigation rate of any industry in America. Efforts at setting liability limits or other approaches to tort reform, unfortunately, follow the idiot's reasoning that the problem is the legal sharks and the legal system. But is it the lawyers who are suing the health care industry into oblivion, or is it the industry's own Customers, very angry Customers who retain lawyers as their agents? Consider the core risk involved: If I take my loved one to the hospital and the wrong blood is transfused, the fury of hell will be unleashed. There is no force that can match a parent's anger over a child lost through dereliction. No effective leader would defend conditions that make Customers want to sue, or allow those conditions to remain in the system. People who get results know that you win most games by going on the offense and scoring points, not just by playing defense. Why do Customers have to force us to perform?

How about a different logic: *Let's do things right so that lawyers don't have a case.* Excellent hospitals find that as they improve their operations, the number of lawsuits they experience annually drops, and so does the size of the average claim settled. Not only do the number of legal problems decline, there is a marked drop-off in complaint letters sent to the CEO. Patients and visitors to the organization sense a greater sense of purpose and effort among staff, and when mistakes happen there seems to be a greater sense of forgiveness because Customers know that staff is trying hard.

Granted that some kind of tort reform is needed, what does it say when hospitals are reported to be spending more on legal liability than they do on hospital training? (To verify this, ask what the numbers are in your organization.) What does it imply about leadership when management allows questionably competent physicians to continue their admitting privileges? Rather than simply taking the position that lawyers are wrong and adopting a bunker mentality, why not go on the offensive and fix the elements in the system that create these problems. Customers won't sue if there is unfailing quality. Think differently. As Plato said, "There are a thousand hacking at the branches of evil for each one striking at the root."

Many health care organizations remain out of touch with their Customers. Although they may mouth Customer service as a value, failing organizations ignore legitimate Customer complaints. Systems are not changed, health care executives often have little contact with patients, and physician issues go unchecked. This is borne out in satisfaction surveys, where a pattern of low scores persists, sometimes for years, with little or no action being taken. It's almost as though the philosophy is "The Customer is right, but not always, and certainly not today."

Prescription. Undertake intense change programs aimed at reducing Customer defection rates and increasing satisfaction scores to a minimal rating of 90 percent "Excellent." Form Strategic Customer Response (SCR) teams on any and all Customer issues to correct problems rapidly. What's the twenty-first century success strategy? Respond!

Failures of Vision

To some degree, leadership's thinking in health care has been in torpor. Rather than rigorously rethinking, health care management has been asleep at the wheel. In the midst of a battlefield, too many leaders have been settling for survival over winning. One sees it in some hospital mergers. The weak join the weak but succeed only in becoming a big, weak organization, not a strong one.

They retain a vain hope that slight adjustments, rather than carving out a new vision, will transform them. Mergers and acquisitions are successful less than half of the time in terms of improving organizational performance. (Discussion on mergers and acquisitions will be found in Chapter Ten under the heading "System Building—A Questionable Track Record."

It's clearly time to rethink the health care organizations' mission, culture, procedures, goals, measures—everything. As one health system leader confided, "No one with responsibility would build health care the way it's currently structured." This is the time for experimentation and generation of new ideas. As another leader said to his management team, "I want you to take this place apart, brick by brick and policy by policy. I want you to create your dreams." Don't do things the way everyone else does. Be contrarian and rebellious. Fight for a new approach. The effective executive is wedded only to results, is aggressive toward that task, and defends nothing in the current system except its sacred values.

Prescription. What's needed now are bold new initiatives for daring new heights of achievement. Shaking people up with the excitement of stretch goal challenges (Chapter Two) and making them realize that what is most to be feared is *not* changing, is a far better approach than hunkering down in a foxhole.

Exorbitant Cost

Any kid running a lemonade stand knows there's a price limit on what Customers will pay for lemonade. Cost reimbursement policies of years past tremendously damaged the hospital industry by creating a mindset that costs needn't be aggressively managed. Rather than being toughened over the years by having to deal with resource limits, the industry was crippled by payers. The result is a lack of experience in dealing with the real world of competition. Health care did not learn how to deal with harsh economic reality as other industries have, and it must rapidly catch up in mastering those skills.

The debate on reimbursement levels is now over. By 1998, 80 percent of employers who offered medical benefits had switched to managed care plans of one sort or another. Washington D.C. and state capitals report that their money trees have died. One could argue that that's not fair to providers, for what is the life of a loved one worth? When health professionals benefit our families, none of us question the *worth* of what's been done, we simply can't *afford* it. What was created in the past was an industry offering a product that literally had priced itself out of the market. And *prices* couldn't be reduced because *costs* were out of control.

As we enter the next century, price increases have slowed due to a low inflation economy, a fortunate outcome but not one resulting from the right management prescriptions. High costs and low quality are the yin and yang of mismanagement. The best assumption for managements to make is that hospitals will have continuously declining resources into the future, and quality will have to be simultaneously improved. Although it may sound paradoxical, the path to decreasing cost is first to increase quality.

Although some managements are rising to the economic challenge, the press continues to report ethical and moral shortcuts taken by other health care executives to make the bottom line: patient dumping ("Two Hospitals Latest to Settle Patient 'Dumping' Cases," 1996), kickbacks to physicians for patient referrals (Snow, 1996), some mergers driven by money instead of mission (Japsen, 1997), billing for tests not done (Pallarito, 1997), fraud (Shinkman, 1996b), and more fraud ("Missouri Hospital Pleads No Contest to Fraud," 1996)—the steady, continuing drumbeat of these sad stories of greed and bad management seem endless. Inevitably, the free market takes its revenge, the lawsuits start (Woodyard, 1997) and health care corporations fall from grace or their executives get terminated or go to jail (Limbacher, 1997). Notwithstanding the outstanding contribution of many thousands of good people within the Columbia-HCA system, the alleged misconduct of a few had disastrous market impact. Opined *Modern Healthcare*: "The stories of fraud and abuse are cascading in the consumer press. The health care industry stands in imminent danger of being lumped in the public mind with the makers of $600 toilet seats, wealthy farmers drawing subsidies, and other perceived treasury raiders. Lawmakers intent on slashing Medicare spending will use this perception to fuel their payment chain saws" ("In Light of Fraud Stories, Industry Should Focus on Reassuring Public," 1997).

Some health care organizations suffer in part because of poor economic stewardship. Organizations on the road to failure eat into their cash reserves, increase their debt burden, borrow from their foundation money, and leave no resources for economic downturns or challenges from competitors. Like the prodigal son, they spend their capital.

Prescription. Instead of covering costs by breaking the law or eliminating staff, management must cut waste in the system: Look for ideas from the staff, not victims to lay off. No organization ever cost-cut their way to excellence. Something more is needed: prescriptions found later in this book.

The Enemies Within

Failing organizations often fail their people or are failed by them. A sour working climate is a response to management inattentiveness. Among the staff this often is expressed by hostile workers or labor conflict, or by the presence of a substantial number of problem employees. The failed strategy of layoffs, and then more layoffs, creates an insecure, demoralized, and increasingly resistant workforce.

There's also the problem of the unqualified. Foreign-trained staff are often both competent and caring—some are not. Skilled people are hard to find and hospitals often hire "warm bodies" because they think "you have to take what you can get." Temporary and part-time workers are often not oriented, have lapsed licenses, or no one checks out their skills.

In one very grinding exposé, the Austin American-Statesman News asserted that military doctors represented a lesser standard. In a long series of articles they alleged that the military system lacked safeguards, that certain physicians were named repeatedly in malpractice suits, that military malpractice cases go unreported to the National Practitioner Data Bank (over 900 incidents were reported in the two-year period 1994–1995), and that the military was letting staff members without medical degrees practice medicine as a way to handle doctor shortages (Carollo and Nesmith, 1977). The private sector is not immune to such charges either, and the question of how to police all professions in health care is proper and critical.

The ranks of management are not immune as the toxic poisons of discontent feed into managerial hypocrisy—leaders who "talk the talk, but don't walk the walk." Managerial flame-out occurs when careers are stultified and aggressive thinking is unrewarded.

Prescription. Remedies include removing unsalvageable performers and working hard at retaining people you don't want to lose (Sherman, 1987). While we're at it, a little job security, job training, and recognition wouldn't hurt. Effective managements know that an unhappy army wins no wars.

Management Myopia

Finally in this sad list is a realization that a lot of very hard-working and well-intentioned leaders in the industry have become disoriented by the endless maze and complexity of modern health care's problems and are punchy from taking so many blows. When one is continuously hammered it's easy to become myopic and no longer see what clearly needs to be done. A *Modern Healthcare* editorial put it this way: "A kind of lethargy is creeping through the healthcare industry as providers, suppliers, and managed-care plans attempt to make sense of the economic, political, and legal bombs that have rocked some of the best-known names in the business. . . . But [this] need not derail an organization's spirit and strategy. Too much doubt can paralyze a company, stopping it from taking the kind of forceful action needed in the dynamic world of healthcare" ("Industry's Troubles Threaten to Trigger Leadership Paralysis," 1998).

Many health care organizations are currently experiencing an identity crisis. When businesses in any industry are undergoing a thorough redefinition demanded by external market forces, leaders often experience a period when they simply don't understand the business. In this rocky phase when the plane spins out of control, executives frantically search for answers, trying various approaches. This problem is now manifesting itself in health care. In its worst manifestation, management often succumbs to a succession of fads, installing a long succession of "programs of the month," and creating change fatigue in the workforce. In your own organization, do managers know what the organization is trying to accomplish? Is there a consistent direction?

Prescription. What is needed is a defined management model of what the business should look like and how it should function.

This model must be tied to a defined winning market strategy—here's where we're going, here's how we will get there—with less zigzagging, more going straight for the goal (see Chapters Two and Six).

There is good news in understanding the difficulties our organizations are experiencing. Because organizational failure is predictable, describable, and fixable, those who want to effect change can be encouraged. This arena of organizational failure is familiar terrain in the field of modern management. We can apply prescriptions that have worked elsewhere. But who will fix it if leaders won't? Who will correct it if leaders do not know how?

The Upward Struggle of Leadership

Now we come to the core of the problem: At the heart of all organizational failure is a failure of management. Whether organizational failure is described in terms of economics, litigation, labor unrest, Customer anger, or interdepartmental conflict, ultimately it's the failure of management. That's what accountability means.

Because the leaders set the standards, it is essential that we understand the nature of this failure. The search for new and better ways of leading our health care organizations requires confronting the elements of leadership thinking that are not working, so we can replace them, and amplify factors that are effective. It will also help if we think of this failure as less a failure of dedicated people and, as we will learn, more a failure of a management approach. It is not blame but understanding that we seek. There is reason to believe that the management approach that worked in the past is largely useless and inapplicable now. A totally changed set of operating needs now requires us to totally rethink the work of management.

All leaders can fail—all leaders can improve. And health care leadership approaches badly need improvement. None want to fail, none set out to fail, but fail they do. When failure involves health care delivery, the results can be tragic for the community, for the jobs lost, for the patients injured or dead, and for reputations lost. The good news is that the idea of continuous improvement applies to what people do as well. What can we do to get on to new and better approaches in the job at hand?

If standards are to be raised in health care generally, they will need to be raised first among the leaders of the industry. No leader asks others to do what she isn't willing to do herself. Current management standards and practices in the industry are too low, in some cases they are unethically low. A related problem is that management practice standards are often unknown or non-uniform within individual organizations, much less in multiunit systems, thus resulting in lower profitability, efficiency, and Customer satisfaction. Make no mistake, our organizations' futures rest in large part on improving management practice standards.

Executive turnover in America's hospitals has shown a consistently high rate approximating 15 percent per year over the last five years, though the rate may be slowing as consolidation slows. In a 1997 study, the rate was 16 percent, the highest in five years, although there was some decline in the year following. In certain states the rate is substantially above the average: Alaska (38 percent), New Mexico (29 percent), Hawaii (28.5 percent), Florida (27 percent), and Virginia (26.7 percent). It can be estimated that 100 percent total top management turnover (presidents and vice presidents) occurred from 1990 through 1997. Even though some of this represented normal transitions (promotions, transfers, consolidations) within the industry, it also included the more negative aspects of termination due to lack of performance capability. Much of the latter represents the unreported failure of individuals and organizations to achieve their goals. Having failed in one location, the failed practitioner often moves on to a new assignment, only to fail again.

From the organization's perspective, boards often feel frustration at removing one executive only to find that their new hire is not substantially better. Search firms operating in the industry report they are receiving an increasing number of requests to submit candidates who do not have hospital background but come from business and industry (ACHE staff, personal communication, 1996).

We are in a period that demands a new leadership profile (I hesitate calling it a style)—one that is power sharing, faster moving, relationship reexamining, goal defining, and behavior rewarding. This new profile will require either new leaders or current leaders moving in new directions. In this period of uncertainty, one thing is certain: Managing by yesterday's rules won't make it. Jack Welch, voted *Fortune's* 1998 Best CEO, is one of the best writers on leadership around, incisive and eloquent. His dicta serve to illustrate the divide that exists between the old and new approaches to leadership in America generally and in the hospital industry particularly (Lowe, 1998).

- I simply dislike the traits that have come to be associated with "managing"—controlling, stifling people, keeping them in the dark, wasting their time on trivia and reports. . . . The word *manager* has too often come to be synonymous with control— cold, uncaring, button-down, passionless. I never associate passion with the word manager, and I've never seen a leader without it.
- One of the things about leadership is that you cannot be a moderate, balanced, thoughtful, careful articulator of policy. You've got to be on the lunatic fringe.
- In an environment where we must have every good idea from every man and woman in the organization, we cannot afford management styles that suppress and intimidate.
- The world of the 1990s and beyond will not belong to "managers" or those who can make the numbers dance. The world will belong to passionate, driven leaders—people who not only have enormous amounts of energy but who can energize those whom they lead.

So, *management* is out, *leadership* is in, but how do I learn leadership? A lot of America's health care leaders haven't been given enough coaching assistance, yet everybody who wins has to go through a process whereby they learn how to win. (General Electric's Management Development Center at Crotonville is legendary.) What can you do quickly by way of management development to make sure your career's in gear? Here are some road rules that may help:

- Go to management seminars outside of the health care industry. Hear how management is conceptualized by the broader management community. If you are a vice president or above, consider doing a concentrated executive program (one to six weeks) at one of the top-flight business schools.

- Read from thought-leading journals like *Fortune* and the *Harvard Business Review.* If it's not in those publications, it's not central to the development of management. There are lots of secondary publications that won't get you as quickly to the core issues. Get them out of your in-basket.
- Create a study group of upwardly mobile friends. Include some management people outside health care. Organize brown-bag lunches for debate following one person's presentation of the core arguments from a new management book.
- Read. Leaders are readers. Where possible, read about the companies and people who are doing something in the real world, the best of breed. A minimum goal would be a book a month. (Lee Iacocca's goal was a book a day.)

Why Good People Falter

Standards in American health care organizations and delivery will rise in direct proportion to the increased quality of health care leaders' performance. The men and women who lead the hospital industry deserve our highest regard. With few exceptions they are people of intellect, courage, and character. But organizational failure and disruption must always be placed at the door of leadership. That's where the buck stops. (For the purposes of this discussion about accountability, leaders are the executives, managers, and supervisors listed on the organizational chart.) When results aren't the best, hard questions have to be asked. To begin working our way out of the forest we don't need criticism, but a critique. Failures, where they have occurred, may be failures of a system of managing rather than those of individual people as leaders. Whatever the causes, we need to understand them if we're to move forward.

Consider this statement from Thomas Teal (1996), former senior editor of the *Harvard Business Review.* He is talking about management mediocrity in all industries, not just health care:

> Look closely at any company in trouble, and you'll probably find that the problem is management. Ask employees about their jobs, and they'll complain about management. Study large corporations, and you'll discover that the biggest barrier to change, innovation, and new ideas is very often management. Make an

inventory of the things that have stifled your own creativity and held back your own career; summarize the critical factors that have stood in the way of your organization's success; name the individuals chiefly responsible for the missed opportunities and bungled projects you yourself have witnessed. Managers will top every list.

There is so much inferior management in the world that some people believe we'd be better off in completely flat organizations with no managers at all. . . . Something about management looks so easy that we watch one anemic performance after another and never doubt that we could succeed where others repeatedly fail. . . .

[T]he troublesome fact is that mediocre management is the norm. This is not because some people are born without the management gene or because the wrong people get promoted or because the system can be manipulated—although all these things happen all the time. The overwhelmingly most common explanation is much simpler: capable management is so extraordinarily difficult that few people look good no matter how hard they try. Most of those lackluster managers we all complain about are doing their *best* to manage well.

Teal's comments are not meant as hypercriticism of people but a statement of a belief that management is mostly about technique. In fact, management is more about personal character and the leadership of people. Organizations do well or ill, based on the quality of the people who run them and whether they are passionately involved and have won the hearts and minds of the people around them. In many of today's hospitals, too few executives see that as their clear focus, and their organizations suffer.

In many ways, the nightmarish existence that hospitals are finally awakening from is a replay of the earlier experience suffered by American business in the 1970s, when industry after industry fell to the onslaught of Japanese companies. Many finger-pointing excuses were offered by American managers as to why their organizations could not compete: too much government regulation, workforce problems, unrealistic quality standards. Analysis showed however that the national failure was a failure of American management (Hayes, 1980).

Lester Thurow, dean of the Massachusetts Institute of Technology Sloan School of Management during that same era, wrote in a *Newsweek* editorial, "When American industries first started to fall behind their foreign competitors, the phenomenon was dismissed as isolated cases of bad luck. The American steel industry just happened to be slow in shifting to oxygen furnaces and continuous casting. Consumer electronics just happened to miss the significance of the transistor. But as the list of industries . . . that have been conquered or need government protection to survive has grown, it has become increasingly obvious that something is systematically wrong with American management" (Thurow, 1981). In the current era, management failure stems from the following five sources.

Questionable Executive Preparation

Most hospital executives received their training in one of America's Master of Hospital Administration (MHA) programs. The set of assumptions and working techniques disseminated there in past years may now be irrelevant in terms of dealing with new realities. The same problem occurred with American MBA programs. Business too often found that MBA-trained leaders were unable to produce results. Indeed, the MBA product led many organizations astray during the last twenty years, when operating concepts failed to compete against companies with very different notions.

During the 1990s, a period when most business school deans were replaced, the press actively told the story of inadequate business preparation in America's MBA programs. *The Wall Street Journal,* reporting on a two-year study by a top-level panel of business school deans, wrote: "MBAs today are merely number-crunchers, ill-prepared to manage. . . . [They have contributed] to America's economic woes . . . [and are not] committed to anything but lofty salaries and titles" (Fuchsberg, 1990). In a *Forbes* report, Richard West, dean of New York University's Stern School of Business, said: "We business schools are going through the agony that organizations go through when they become producer-driven. To a significant degree, we lost sight of our Customers—students and corporations" (Linden, Brennan, and Lane, 1992). And *Fortune* wrote: "Business education's current plunge into self-analysis is the deepest in thirty years, prompted by . . . increasing complaints from companies about the usefulness of MBAs. . . . The pressure on the nation's 700-plus business schools to improve their products is high" (O'Reilly, 1994).

Have hospital executives been as inadequately prepared as their business counterparts? Have MHA programs kept up with the revolutionary changes occurring in MBA programs? Assessing the adequacy of MHA programs or continuing professional development on the job, although beyond the scope of this book, is an area that needs examining. Something is wrong in leadership, either in the selection of the people entering the profession, their academic preparation, or the mentoring they receive.

Of course this whole discussion is simply meant to encourage the return of hospital administration studies to the fold of management where it belongs. Historically, the rise of public administration and hospital administration programs was a reaction against business management in the years of the Great Depression. There was hostility against business and business executives of that era, and a way to protect the image of government and health care organizations was to give their pursuits a different name, a reaction of political correctness (Drucker, 1998). But management is management, and in the modern era, being separated or divorced from the mainstream of management thought has a damaging effect on the evolution of health care organizations. Leaders must think outside the narrow confines of their particular industry and embrace tools and techniques that have proven effective elsewhere.

No one questions the desire of health leaders to do a good job. But wanting to do well may not be enough. One also has to know how to do it right. Our new health care organizations require a new leadership, and this ultimately means either new or retrained, revitalized, and rededicated leaders. It's been said that you can't win with losers, and the untrained and undertrained are a liability on any battlefield. This question is key to any standards discussion, for it is the leaders who set the standard.

Lack of Appropriate Mentors

A comparison of executive careers in business with those in health care show a number of remarkable differences in personality type, early life history, academic preparation, and other factors. In business, a manager's mentors have typically risen through a hierarchy of tough competitors, have many years of experience in cost-driven and market-driven industries, have operated with tough cultural guidelines of what to do, and have the sophisticated work systems necessary to do their work. By contrast, today's health care leaders have often been mentored by executives of a bygone era who had little competitive experience, were computer illiterate, and showed a "good old boy" naivete about how to run a business. This is not to demean people, for we are all the byproduct of our conditioning. As one management veteran said, "I was the victim of a series of accidents, as are we all." By lack of experience, health care mentors were often unable to pass on presently needed skills.

It wasn't that long ago in health care that competition was considered "naughty" and *profit* a dirty word. Even today's widespread lag in computer linkages among departments, internally, and with physicians and clinics, externally, bespeaks yesterday's failure to comprehend the need to embrace technological change. As one reads the departure statements of one hospital executive after another, many still in their forties and fifties, one realizes a numbing sameness to them: They are leaving by "choice" or "mutual decision"; they have no immediate plans for what they will do next; and when a reaction comment can be obtained, it is usually an observation that the job had become "less fun." One wonders whether these folks might not have been in a different place had their mentoring and experience been different.

Tough times require tough and competent leadership. There is nothing wrong with our organizations that can't be fixed by a new infusion of skills needed for the task and the committed energy of those who want to win the day. This is a transitional problem that is working its way through the industry as new thinking enters and the old is forced out. Much of this transition in thinking is simply a matter of learning new approaches on the part of leaders in place. Unfortunately, the departure of those who do not know how to lead, and are unwilling to master the new approaches, will be painful but necessary.

Culture Wars

As systems have emerged, the inevitable tending to one's career interests requires establishing new communication networks and a lot of political interfacing. Where will I end up in this new organization? Who will sponsor me now? On what side of issues should

I lean? What coalitions should I build? This normal human political behavior is lamentable only because it takes so much time and distracts from the real work of these leaders.

Many CEOs have been caught up in various system assignments, serving on special committees and task forces. This system activity siphons away a lot of attention needed by the business units. In the meantime, who's minding the store? During this period, individual organizational entities continue to languish, decisions are delayed, work isn't done, and problems escalate. This slowdown in organizational adaptation, in an organization type already behind in its business evolution, exacerbates the problem.

The problems within new system consolidations become even worse with the inevitable variances in cultures and traditions. Instead of designing the new culture, executives skirmish over their differences, each seeing the battlefield in the light of their past experience and conditioning. The psychological energy drain and its related business costs are incalculable.

A Failure of Expectations

Perhaps the greatest trap for current leaders is not staying focused on higher standards and greater expectation of improved organization performance. To help avoid that problem, here's a checklist, a risk list, to alert you of where leaders must be careful not to fail. Check off those that may apply to your situation. Leaders can fail by

- Not understanding that higher standards offer competitive advantage.
- Not recognizing that existing standards and quality management approaches have proved to be not inappropriate but insufficient in dozens of patient misadventures per hospital per year.
- Accepting a status quo effort, going through the motions of quality management, even though out-of-control performances continue to occur—a classic example of what Edwards Deming called the "fallacy of best efforts."
- Not breaking out of the cookie cutter, "me-too" mentality. Rather than thinking like entrepreneurial, independent

business leaders, who would have taken a new tack when it became clear old approaches were stillborn, they continue doing what isn't working.

- Maintaining a country club culture of special privileges for the elite, and continuing a style of nonstructured, nonspecific direction, even though times call for real marching orders.
- Tolerating staff abuse, interdepartmental conflict, and turf wars rather than building a cohesive and cooperative team.
- Maintaining an out-of-touch, remote-control management style (reading reports instead of talking to people on the floor). When endless committee meetings and memos fail to produce results, don't just hold even more meetings, or issue more memos.
- Being subverted by the old existing system—leaders find themselves sinking into the quicksand and becoming part of the problem, not part of the solution.
- Approaching corrective efforts in a disjointed fashion. Rather than coordinating efforts, or staying with one set of priorities, change is attempted on a piecemeal basis, often with departments not even knowing about changes that will affect them until notified shortly before implementation.

In the leadership vacuum that emerges in these situations, consultants tend to enter the play. The hospital industry has become a consultant's dream. The word is out in the consulting industry that hospitals will buy anything. Said one consultant, "We knew they'd have a high failure rate with TQM, but you've got to sell what the market demands. When that wave was pretty much over, we ramped up to do reengineering, knowing it was going to go down the same path." Consequently, programs with good conceptual content but little chance of survival in the often nonreceptive culture of hospitals are heavily marketed and eagerly bought, only to be replaced by the next wave of equally dubious projects. Not only are financial resources bled out by an unholy alliance of inept executives and unscrupulous consultants, but with each successive program the organization becomes more exhausted, change fatigued, and cynical.

Noted organization psychologist Dr. Mark Silber (personal communication) succinctly described the sickened organization that results from a malpracticing management: "Vaguely defined outputs from an organization in a state of confused authority distribution, emanating from a placid centralization of nondirection, converging into disjointed efforts toward crisis fire fighting, reacted to by on-the-job-retirees with decreasing resources."

A Failure of Ethics

The twin forces of competition and greed have been a breeding ground for faulty thinking on the part of some in management. In the new and still undefined world of emerging health care management, the internal compass has often not pointed true north. Stories of questionable billing practices, fraud, and conflicts of interest have abounded in the nation's press. These things didn't just happen by mistake—every one of these cockeyed ideas was actually approved. People sat down in meetings, discussed these items, and made a decision.

Such incidents are not representative of the overwhelming majority of health care leaders whose personal and business standards are above reproach, but they signal that the opportunity of a free marketplace, so essential for the future progress of the industry, brings with it new risks. Defining and enforcing standards of ethical conduct is an essential activity for individuals, organizations, and the health care industry. As with the errors made in business and the military in recent years, these problems suggest that efforts at correction need to be made. Courses in ethics, corporate policies regarding conduct standards and conflicts of interest, and emphasis of values-centered management will be part of the solution. A drift in principle always leads to a drift in organizational performance. As the health care industry moves forward, the essential question of how fit its leadership is to lead will remain active and central.

Needed: A New Management Team

After describing organizational failure and laying the responsibility at the doorstep of top leaders, the question of what will be needed to change our organizations is still not adequately answered. Executives, no matter how skilled, cannot do it by themselves: An effective management team has to be part of the answer.

Hospital managers are typically promoted from their technical specialties, most often without any assessment procedure that would measure their capability to manage. The fallacy is to take the best technical worker and make him a manager. This causes double jeopardy: In addition to losing its best technician, the organization may have gained only a mediocre manager. This questionable selection procedure is compounded by a starved management development environment that fails to nurture or grow the skills necessary for managerial work. The organizational structure then keeps people in departmental isolation, thus avoiding the formation of anything remotely resembling a team.

One obvious prescription is to provide a strong management development program for all managers. This shouldn't be a lightweight course that talks about topics in management without providing impetus and skills for changing the organization. Rather, it should show managers how to do their job, then require them to go back into the organization and change it to fit those better approaches. Unless the ability to discuss and act on the organization's problems is part of the course work, the educational effort will be insufficient. Team bonding occurs when management works together to make change.

An example of how education of leaders can help change organizational behavior is to do an assessment of each manager's approach to his job and how that approach affects the organization as a whole. I have used a testing inventory known as the Leadership Opinion Questionnaire over the years to measure hospital teams. Under this model, *leadership* is defined simply as "the ability to get followers." This means that someone can have an organizational title, but if people do not willingly follow that person but only comply with orders, the person is only a figurehead, not a leader. Conversely, someone without a position of authority over others may represent others' interests to the extent that allegiance is willingly given. Informal group leaders are often examples of this.

The Leadership Opinion Questionnaire (Fleishman, 1989) measures the two factors found to be most critical in getting positive performance from followers—*Consideration* (is caring, concerned; is a two-way communicator; listens well; asks for ideas; goes to bat, is supportive; establishes rapport, relationship; shows how, is a developer; celebrates wins, is a rewarder) and *Structure* (sets work goals; sets deadlines; has high expectations; has high standards of performance; demands results and effort; makes tough decisions; sets example, lives standards; pushes to do more, encourages). These are the requisite requirements that followers need from leaders if the leader's power is to be effective.

For a leader to be effective, at least medium and preferably high scores are needed on both factors. A leader who is high on consideration but low on structure creates a "country club" world with few demands. Conversely, a leader who is high in structure but low in consideration would be seen as a dictator.

In Figure 1.1 these scores have been plotted for a client hospital via an old and reliable tool known as the Managerial Grid. This allows the team to see how their individual scores on consideration (labeled *Concern for People* on the grid) and structure (labeled *Concern for Production*) translate into organizational behavior. Figure 1.1 shows individual scores and the average score, which is considered the descriptor point for how the organization will perform.

Five areas of the grid are described generally to show how the organization performs based on the composite attitudes being expressed by the management team:

- Impoverished: Little concern for people or in getting the work out. Such organizations are dead or dying. Theoretically possible, but they don't last long.
- Country Club: A nice set of folks, but not much work getting done. Typical of some academic environments or other places where you don't have to worry about paying the light bill.
- Task: Extreme examples would have been the American slave system or child labor. Work environments that forget people may tend toward unionization—a troubling element resurging in the hospital industry.
- Middle Road: The organization shows moderate amounts of people and work orientation, muddles through, and is an average performer.
- Team: Things really cook, a lot is getting done; people are working hard and having a good time. This is the area of excellent organizations—a competitor's worst nightmare.

Figure 1.1. A Management Team on the Managerial Grid.

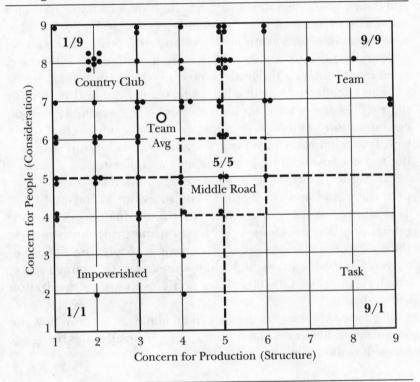

Source: Blake and Mouton, (1964) 1994.

Although theoretically a hospital might achieve a composite score at any one of the eighty-one intersection points, in reality most organizations' composite scores are found inside an ellipse with end points at 1/1 and 9/9. Economics don't permit many organizations to exist anywhere near a 1/9, and labor law pretty much forbids 9/1 treatment of people.

Figure 1.1 illustrates a common pattern we've found among hospital management teams. It indicates a group of people positively oriented toward human values but weaker in their orientation toward getting the work out. Such groups will typically start meetings late, wait for orders rather than initiate projects, miss deadlines, have no written quarterly work plans. Their goals will be unclear, have few outcomes measures, and have disappointing results. Because this approach lacks control over work, a great deal of crisis firefighting typically results. This lack of structure tends to tolerate poor performance in problem workers who seem to multiply under this leadership. Executives often complain that their managers seem to duck accountability, demonstrate undesirable resistance (usually through passive noncompliance), and show a lack of follow through and urgency with problems. Does any of this sound familiar?

Notice also the spread in scores among the individuals. This represents a problem with too much variance resulting from widely different views of how the managerial job should be done, and it erodes team functioning. It is not possible, and probably not desirable, to have everybody at the same point on the grid, but what is important is to have a smaller amount of variance and a general mindset that both high consideration and high structure should be pursued.

These scores are from an actual client assessment. After a year of management development, the insertion of more structured management procedures, and some turnover, a retest of the team showed that the combined average had moved into the Team quadrant. As a consequence, business performance showed marked improvement. Another approach to the low structure problem may be to look for high structure characteristics in new management hires.

Beyond being careful about selecting people who will have the capabilities for the tasks of management, what can be done with incumbent managers? The goal for the organization is to move the management team's approach to managing into the Team quadrant by increasing their orientation to the structure component of their job. For most managers, these problems can be overcome through intensive management development and by instituting a housewide systematic approach to managing that focuses on structural procedures. Although experience has shown that a few managers will not be able to make these transitions, most can. And the real kicker is that improvement in business performance directly results from this movement to a greater structure orientation.

A Standardized Management System

Professions are professions because they follow a set of best practices—the procedures and practices known to achieve desired outcomes. Management is one of the few occupations in health care that has not rigorously defined how to do its job. It is not standardized, and therefore not fully a profession. The result is that most managers pick up some ideas here and there, or imitate their boss's or peers' habits, whether good or ill. In most organizations what results is a patchwork of various and often conflicting approaches to management. Endless hours are wasted, and careers ruined, because there is no common approach to getting the job done that all can agree on. A past challenge for professional management has been to define what the best practice truths and procedures are. Those are now known but still widely unapplied in health care. The paucity of a defined way of doing the tasks of management will retard the organizational progress needed by the industry. Standards and standardization must come to managing.

Ironically, the approaches to effective management are well known. They simply need to be installed. To assist the industry, we developed a tool called MANSYS, the Integrated Management System, which we have made available at our Internet site (www. ManagementHouse.com). It is a working toolset of the techniques, forms, and procedures for getting work done and leading people. Appendix A shows the table of contents and indicates what is needed to get everybody on the team operating in concert. Not only do these approaches reduce the lack of structure problem, but they increase team feeling by creating a sense of unified direction and command.

A management system is a key ingredient when it comes to the standards issues. Define the standard of management practice, get the results it brings, and move on to the work of improving organizational performance.

A New Heart and a New Mind

I am a little uncomfortable in describing the needed improvements in health care leadership in the terms used thus far. Something more is called for—the attitude of winning. Those who lead know that the heart of a champion must be summoned forth. In my work with thousands of managers over the last thirty years I have constantly marveled at the greatness and the potential that lies inside most people, and how rarely leaders ask people to function at this level.

How do you inspire people to want greatness? I don't know that you can. What I do know is that if you arrange an entire management team in a circle, with no furniture in between them, and go around the circle and ask each person to say what their dream is for their job life, for the place in which they are spending their life, you get some great and moving statements. In that arrangement ask them whether they think it is possible to move from the current level of performance to the mountain top. Ask them if they have what it takes to do the impossible. In an hour or so you'll know the mettle of their spirit. My prediction is that you may walk out feeling chagrined that you did not know what they have been willing and wanting to do for years but nobody in leadership ever asked of them.

Conclusion

This chapter has examined the changes necessary for leadership to make in its approach to managing people and work if the list of changes needed by the health care industry is to succeed. Because leadership is always by example, we have started the process of working for change by introspectively revisiting the touchstones of superior managing. The formation of a new managing approach will be crucial for the success that is there for the taking. In the next chapter we will find out that raising standards is a question that must be worked out in relationship to what the market requires. Standards raised in directions the market isn't interested in would be a mistake. Reaching for the stars is part of raising standards, but we need to make sure we're heading somewhere in the universe that the market is interested in going.

Work-Out Session

1. In MANSYS, the Management System, we suggest that each person write out their own mission statement. What is the

purpose of your life and career at work? What are you willing to dedicate yourself to? What do you want to achieve for your people, your department, your profession, your patient? What do you want for you?

2. List the organizational or departmental performance problems that concern you. Which are simply operational to-do's? Which are indications of serious organization dry rot?

3. Identify from the organization failure profile the top three areas where you think your organization needs improvement:
   Quality control
   Reining in bureaucracy
   Keeping in touch with Customers
   Failures of vision
   Costs out of control
   Morale

4. Identify from the leadership failure profile two areas where the management team needs to pay closer attention.
   Executive preparation
   Appropriate mentors
   Rising above the culture war concept
   Meeting expectations
   Heightened ethical awareness
   A new leadership team and approach to managing
   A new management system

Chapter Two

The Strategy-Standards Equation

A salesman traveling down the highway chances on a farm where the buildings, trees, corral posts, and mailbox are covered with hundreds of targets. Smack-dab in the center of each target is a single bullet hole. Unbelievable! Hundreds of bull's eyes and no misses. He screeches to a halt, bangs on the farmer's door, and asks, "How do you do it? What's the secret to being such a great marksman?"

The farmer responds. "Well, I've got this trusty carbine. Hand load the ammunition myself. Got a twenty-power sight on it. Lots of experience, too, that sure helps. I put a shell in the chamber, lock the bolt down, and gently squeeze off a shot. Now, wherever that bullet hits, I just take a can of paint and a brush, and paint me a target!"

It's easy when you know the secret. The unfortunate truth is that too many health care organizations operate without targets. That statement is easily tested by asking managers and staff what their targets are. Often no one knows. At the end of the year—surprise! We didn't get where we wanted to go. If standards are to be elevated in American health care, we had better clarify where we're headed or the direction we take is not likely to be the correct one.

This chapter spotlights three of the more exciting developments in modern management and shows how they can interact synergistically to produce better results in how health care organizations perform. These themes—market positioning, stretch goals, and scorecarding—are essential for strategic direction yet are rarely found in the health industry. Taken together, these elements form an exciting new dynamic and provide a more certain way to manage the organization for the challenges ahead:

- *Market positioning that wins.* Organizations take certain positions relative to their market; that is, they are seen as providing services in a particular way by their market. But only some positions are winning ones. How should the twenty-first century health care organization align itself with the new market reality of long-term resource scarcity in a managed care environment? How do market leaders discipline themselves to fit the market?

- *Goals that drive performance.* Organizations without goals don't tend to achieve very much. Winning organizations follow a particular approach to goal setting and reward. Not only must goals be clarified in this era of chaos and drift, but they must be made challenging and realistic to the organization's members.

- *Measures that make better management possible.* Measures tell us where we are now and help us determine whether efforts to improve are moving in the right direction. What new measures are needed to direct and renew our organizations? How can measures be used to guide upstream factors that produce positive performance rather than looking at after-the-fact, downstream financial facts?

Raising standards begins with getting the organization oriented to where it has to go in terms of its overall performance. Overall performance is always tied to market requirements. More discrete standards concerns such as clinical performance, information systems upgrading, or personnel issues have little chance of success if the larger picture isn't clarified right at the start. And the big picture we're shooting for is world-class organizational performance, within which is found world-class practices and individual behaviors.

Get Right with the Market

While health care struggles to find the right combination to meet the needs of a changing market, a copycat atmosphere has developed in which certain prescriptions are being accepted wholesale without a lot of rigorous thought. Consolidation into chains, or integration of services, may sometimes be good approaches. The concern is not whether these ideas should be considered or embraced where appropriate. The concern is that primary and better approaches to organizational performance are being omitted, an omission that may cause secondary strategies like consolidation or integration to fail.

Studies of successful organizations show clearly that the first part of any market strategy must be *proper positioning relative to market requirements*. Unless a hospital or health care system provides the market with what it wants, it will surely fail. It either provides what is wanted or is surpassed by others who will. This first law of fitting the organization to the market has been broken repeatedly. The landscape is littered with dead hospitals and "systems" that have come and gone, either consumed by those who were smarter or, more accurately stated, by those who had the discipline to obey the first law. Said B. C. Forbes, founder of *Forbes* and keen observer of the rise and fall of organizations: "If you don't drive your business, you will be driven out of business. The prize is for the alert, for the enterprising, for the farsighted, for the energized, for those quick to adapt themselves and their organization to new and changing conditions."

"New and changing conditions" are certainly in evidence in health care, particularly the tough demands for better cost, quality, and service. This has resulted in an environment in which extreme competition prevails for many organizations. Are there approaches that have been found to work in other industries that might provide benchmark guidance as to what should be done in this new environment?

Researchers have discovered that organizations that win in the marketplace make a conscious decision to be one of three kinds of providers ("How Market Leaders Keep Their Edge," 1995). These three ways to win succeed because they represent a good fit or alignment with market variables that management can never control, only exploit. It is important to understand that hospitals can improve their survivability by moving to one of these safer positions precisely because these three positions represent defensibility. In a competitive environment, the question isn't whether the organization will come under attack but whether it is in a defensible position when it is attacked. Standardization of best practices is defined differently based on the market position the organization takes. Hence, this question has to be resolved prior to making decisions regarding standards and standardization.

Porter's Generic Strategies Model

Michael Porter of the Harvard Business School began a revolution in market thinking with his books on *Competitive Strategy* and *Competitive Advantage* (Porter, 1998a, 1998b). He is a leading proponent of correct market positioning as a predictor of organizational success. Porter identifies three strategies around which an organization can build its core competencies:

1. Low cost: Achieve overall low-cost leadership against competitors. Low cost makes low price possible and is suitable to mass markets.
2. Differentiation: Products are differentiated in ways valuable to select Customers, usually at a high-end cost. These are usually luxury items or items aimed at those for whom cost is secondary.
3. Focus: Focus on specific niche markets for growth by offering highly specialized products that appeal to a market segment.

Porter argues that an organization can enhance its competitive positioning by performing key internal activities in the value chain at a lower cost or better than its competitors. The value-chain approach identifies primary and secondary activities. *Primary activities* include production, marketing, logistics, and after-sale functions. *Secondary activities* are support processes to primary activities. These include firm infrastructure, human resource management, technology development, and procurement. The ultimate purpose of the firm is to add as much Customer "value" as it can to each of the primary activities.

Let's examine briefly how these three strategies work to see which might be appropriate to the "average" health care provider.

Win Through Cost: The Managed Care Opportunity

Winning through cost allows an organization to win in its pricing. Hospitals become terrified of the managed care environment because they know their cost structures are out of control. Feeling victimized by managed care contracts, they turn to self-mutilation (staff reductions) or sacrifice their future (cut off capital investment). The key to winning in the cost game is to achieve *Operational Excellence*. Because *low cost* is not inspiring as a phrase to rally people around, we have used *Operational Excellence* as a more inclusive and motivating term.

Operational Excellence means no waste of resources and no redo of work. It means using best practice methods and having real purchasing control. It means that the organization *must* execute its core work processes extremely well, with real precision and attention to detail, and make every shot count in terms of efficient use of resources. Some examples are Wal-Mart and Ford's Taurus, which are both lower priced, volume leaders in their respective industries.

The low-cost or Operational Excellence strategy does not mean a cheap or shoddy product. To succeed, quality must be acceptably high, and the other elements of Customer connection and service must be adequate. But cost, the first variable in the cost-quality-service triad, must be met if the objective is to create a product affordable to all.

Practicing cost leadership involves placing great emphasis on efficiency in all organizational activities to reduce the overall costs of products delivered to Customers. A generic low-cost leadership strategy only works effectively when the organization can provide products and/or services at a cost lower than the competition's.

K Mart tried to function as the low-cost provider, but the closing of hundreds of K Mart stores and near bankruptcy in 1997 attested to a failure of execution. For example, although K Mart duplicated the Wal-Mart greeter, Customers could detect differences in selection and training in the quality of that first impression. Many other subtle differences, some seen, some unseen by Customers, accounted for the success of Wal-Mart as a "category killer." The bottom-line lesson: Success is a combination of the right market strategy and execution of that strategy.

Because this strategy inevitably means low profit margins, it requires that the organization goes for market share to build profit volume. Arguably, this is difficult when the market is semi-controlled by payers, but patients and payers alike will eventually respond to favorable price and quality outcomes. Unfortunately, some health care providers resemble the old salesman who was lamenting that he was losing money on every sale. His friend said, "That's bad." The salesman replied, "No, that's good. I make up for it in volume!" Volume can compensate for lower margins, but only if proper and efficient execution is possible. The organization that can achieve high performance in Operational Excellence can possibly win a price war whereas others cannot. For example, because Wal-Mart controls pilferage by Customers and Associates better than K Mart, an additional 2 percent profit falls to the bottom line that gives them room to compete more aggressively on price. Whenever Wal-Mart does, K Mart hemorrhages red ink.

Operational Excellence requires the following steps to establishing cost leadership:

- Create or distribute only good quality products
- Draw advantages from many sources, including suppliers and Customers
- Study the competition
- Make cost or value a part of corporate culture

Hospitals must build their cost leadership position on these steps. The challenge is to furnish the Customer with a quality service using a multitude of competitive advantages, low-cost suppliers, and an extremely efficient delivery system. The health care organization must incorporate cost leadership as part of its mission and culture. The message to the Customer stresses value and unfailing quality. Customers do not equate a value price with poor quality, for they know that quality is associated with input and process variables that result in high-tech, high-touch care. That result can be achieved by doing things better and more efficiently, and by focusing on the true needs of Customers.

Win with Differentiation: High-End Products and Services

A *differentiation* strategy involves delivering products or services that are different from the product mix of the competition. Differentiated products are often marketed at premium prices to balance the added costs associated with differentiation. This strategy creates higher profit margins than Operational Excellence but trades away the ability to offer it to a mass market. A potential risk associated with this strategy is that consumers may not perceive the product or service as differentiated. For example, is an appendectomy or bypass here better than an appendectomy or bypass there? Can you back the answer up statistically, not just in marketing language?

Under this approach an organization must differentiate itself so it's perceived as significantly better in quality, design, service, brand name, or reputation. Some familiar examples outside health care are Nordstrom and Lexus. To some degree the "high-end" may be more perception than reality, since a number of the clothing brands at Nordstrom may be carried by other retailers as well. But it is the image or the quality of interaction from Nordstrom's superior sales staff that makes the total buying experience one that is perceived as more elegant. In the case of Lexus, the product quality can be clearly demonstrated as superior with the added plus that it is more affordable than many other luxury contenders.

The opportunity associated with being a high-end provider is that it allows charging a higher than average price that Customers are often willing to pay. For people who can afford to pay, this strategy can be a winner. The problem for health care providers is there aren't many managed care contractors interested in buying this argument, so it's a poor strategy to pursue for the majority of the market. It can be a winner for those who can afford to pay.

Win Through Focus: Unique Offerings

Under this market position strategy, an organization focuses on particular Customers, geographic areas, distribution channels, or service lines not exploited by others. The pursuit of niche markets can work when the organization's offerings are unique and where it can be dominant with those who can afford them. Examples are L. L. Bean and the Hummer utility vehicle. Like high-end providers, the unique provider always charges more but must exchange that for smaller markets and higher product or marketing costs. Although Arnold Schwarzenegger may drive a Hummer, it's possible that no one you know personally does.

Michael Porter argues that a focus strategy is actually a mix of the two earlier generic strategies. It focuses on cost leadership and product differentiation simultaneously in one particular market segment, or niche. In health care, certain specialized services (genetic counseling) or surgical specialties (organ transplants) are examples of unique offerings. A difficulty may arise when a niche service line is tied to the rest of the organization, which is pursuing an Operational Excellence strategy. If a focus strategy is to be pursued for certain services, consideration should be given to spinning these off to another setting with different decision makers and organizational constraints. (This is Regina Herzlinger's argument for focused factories in health care, which is discussed later in this book.)

Don't Dabble in Multiple Positions

Simply picking a market position is not enough. To win, an organization must "pick and stick." The evidence strongly suggests that organizations who rigorously stay within their defined market strategy will win. Treacy and Wiersmas (1997) reported in *The Discipline of Market Leaders* that organizations who led and dominated their markets displayed organizational behaviors they referred to as *discipline*. The discipline aspect of market positioning is to *avoid dabbling* in other approaches. These authors found that it was impossible to establish market leadership by trying to be in the no-man's land between these three successful positions. Examples would include Montgomery Ward in retailing or Oldsmobile in automobiles. Neither of these organizations are known for low cost, being best in their class, or offering something special and unique. Both flounder on the edges of their markets, having attained the mediocrity associated with organizations without the discipline to get into alignment with their markets. Sears advertises special sales weekly (low-cost dabbling), whereas Wal-Mart, with "every-day low prices," advertises only once a month. The 75 percent of advertising cost saved falls to Wal-Mart's bottom line. In Oldsmobile's case, discussions have repeatedly been held within GM as to whether the division should be phased out, since it has shown steadily declining market share for over a decade.

In the real world of organizational decision making, there's always someone wanting to make a case to add this luxury service or that unique offering. To try to make the organization all things to all people is a continual temptation. These newly proposed offerings always have a certain logic and attractiveness to them, and there's never a shortage of advocates. Winning organizations are those that have learned the discipline of staying with their business core. Although difficult to do, it is increasingly necessary in an age of tight resources. The reader who may be generally persuaded by the logic of an Operational Excellence strategy may begin to feel queasy over the suggestion that exceptions to its discipline are ill advised. Individual decision makers must call it as they see it, but beware of an undisciplined approach to the market. *Pick and stick* with only one strategy, even though that may seem difficult politically and organizationally.

Organizations successful in the pursuit of a single disciplined market-positioning strategy report that the organization must dedicate itself to the idea of creating breakthrough performance —to be "best in class," not just another contender in its selected arena. Why? Only by being not just in a clearly targeted market position but also really great at it can the organization create for itself a *defensible market position*. Defensibility provides a far more certain world in which to operate.

One solution for multiunit systems may be to create separate divisions in which these three, very different, market strategies can be isolated—a condition for ultimate success. Under that scenario, units trying to provide low-cost services can pursue that agenda and units pursuing special service strategies with their associated higher cost can be grouped away from the elements necessary for Operational Excellence.

For our purposes the argument for Operational Excellence has to be left there. Marketing professionals and chief executives may not be entirely satisfied with my explanations or suggested limitations on organizational involvement—they may well want to dabble. But based on my discussions with health care leaders I believe there is more agreement than disagreement on these features and a belief that some movement in the direction I have espoused is necessary.

Features of Operational Excellence

Operational Excellence is the market position that best fits the managed care imperative to control cost, quality, and Customer satisfaction. What are some of the features that define it? And what would a health care organization have to do to achieve it?

- Deliver: The output from the organization must be a package that contains three elements—great quality, affordable price, and ease of use. What is guaranteed is a low price, hassle-free service, and a standardized product.
- Goal: Customer loyalty (retention) means repeat business, positive word of mouth in the community, and the ability to attract new Customers. This can be achieved only if the organization can exceed and stay ahead of continuously rising Customer expectations. It also means there are limits in terms of the amount of service innovations or degree of tailoring provided to Customers. Remember, a standardized excellent product at a low price requires that we stick with the core competency and not dabble.
- Business processes: Work must be optimized. That requires *discontinuous improvement,* that is, throwing out all the stuff that produces nothing for Customers, refining aggressively the flow of work, streamlining supply chains, and sticking to provision of basic core services to minimize cost and reduce Customer hassles.
- Structure: Organizational structure should have as few levels and departments as possible. Operations must be standardized and simplified, tightly controlled, and centrally planned or reviewed. This means few low-level decisions in terms of exceptions from a highly defined set of operations combined with a lot of upward input on improvements that result in an ever-changing and better model.
- Management systems: The ideal is best described as results-driven as opposed to the endlessly meeting-minded hospital world that is fast disappearing. Systems are highly integrated (lots of computerization) and reliable (systems, not people, catch glitches such as medication errors), transactions are high-speed (waiting times decline), and compliance is achieved with measured operational norms and procedures (internal controls, not external inspections).
- Culture: The organization rewards efficiency, abhors waste, and acts with machine-like predictability. Everybody knows what they are supposed to do and what is expected of every position. Training is constant. The organization is aggressive in stealing ideas and leapfrogging its competition. It stays

ahead of the pack at all times and focuses on being quick to market, whether in offering new services or in handling today's patient call light.

As a management educator I have tried to simplify the explanation of the Operational Excellence strategy so that it can be quickly expressed and understood. Under my model, Operational Excellence contains the four primary elements of high satisfaction, high quality, low cost, and best people (Figure 2.1). The purpose of boiling this down to a few phrases is to create a picture that staff can understand.

The Balanced Scorecard

Once a clear commitment and expression of market positioning has been decided, the organization is ready to begin to manage with a powerful tool called the balanced scorecard (Kaplan and Norton, 1992, 1993, 1996). Several years ago we began work on a set of measures that would assess performance on each of management's Key Results Areas (KRAs)—customer satisfaction, quality,

Figure 2.1. Operational Excellence Strategy.

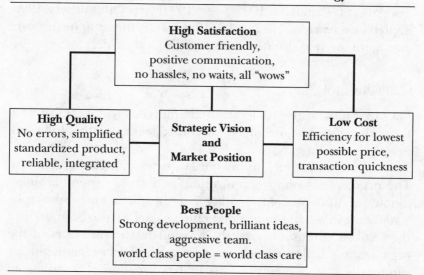

High Satisfaction
Customer friendly,
positive communication,
no hassles, no waits, all "wows"

High Quality
No errors, simplified
standardized product,
reliable, integrated

**Strategic Vision
and
Market Position**

Low Cost
Efficiency for lowest
possible price,
transaction quickness

Best People
Strong development, brilliant ideas,
aggressive team.
world class people = world class care

people growth, organizational climate, innovation, productivity, and economics (Sherman, 1993). This tool was a needed response to the tyranny of financial measures that were throwing decision makers into a one-sided view of the organization, for what one measures often determines how one conceptualizes the management job (Kaplan, 1991).

The idea of finding and using other measures to better gauge the full dynamic of organizational functioning, rather than relying simply on financial controls, has been growing. According to a study by the Institute of Management Accountants, 64 percent of U.S. companies were by 1997 experimenting with or using some sort of new organizational performance management system (Kurtzman, 1997). Indeed, the movement toward new measures represents a true metrics revolution in the private sector ("Counting What Counts," 1997).

By identifying the true performance drivers of the business (for example, Customer satisfaction, innovation, quality indicators), and validating their impact on subsequent economic performance, management can tell exactly where it needs effort and redirection. Using our earlier work of attempting to create a KRA measures matrix, we added to it the related and parallel thinking of other practitioners who had been attempting not only to expand management measures but also to tie that to empowering workers (Caggiano, 1994; Case, 1994; Greer and others, 1992; Kaplan and Norton, 1992, 1993, 1996). In rethinking health care management, it is also necessary to rethink measures.

Using the Tool

Let's first look at the tool and then analyze why it works so well. Properly used, the balanced scorecard achieves the following practical outcomes:

1. Summarizes various mission, vision, and values statements. The problem for many organizations is that they spend an inordinate amount of time creating lengthy plans and philosophy statements in a well-intentioned effort to define the business, but then fail in communicating their vision to the members of the organization. Unless this information can be concisely and quickly summarized, it is useless in providing direction. The balanced

scorecard accomplishes this summary of various mission and vision statements on a single sheet of paper (see Figure 2.2). Since the lengthy discussions to create this thinking have already taken place in most health care organizations, a wordsmith or managerial team can usually extract the key elements from existing documents for the one-page summary.

Executive feedback. In our developmental work with the tool we involved a group of thirty-five health care executives to advise us as they implemented and evaluated each element of the scorecard. They agreed unanimously that a concise summary of the

Figure 2.2. Organization Mission and Philosophy.

Fantastic Memorial Hospital

Who are we?   We're needed and important

We are an army of 3000 highly skilled health professionals who intend to make a greater impact on the health of the communities we serve. We are the oldest and best hospital in the state.

What's our mission?   What we're here to do

To aggressively care for the health needs of our communities, to move rapidly and comprehensively forward in implementing new treatment and prevention approaches, and to improve the quality of life for our Customers

What's our vision?   How we will change the world

We intend to become the premiere hospital in our region and to materially change and improve how health care is delivered. We will become one of the nation's top 100 hospitals and a recognized leader and example to others.

What are our beliefs?   How we will always act

Customer – Always first
Actions – Speak louder than words
Respect — The golden rule
Excellence – In all that we do

What are our goals?   How we will succeed

We must achieve four essential goals: high satisfaction, high quality, low cost, and best people. We will boldly pursue specific objectives and project initiatives, measure how we're doing, and create our future. Each team is empowered to decide what work must be done to contribute to these goals and win.

mission information was essential, and that this page should convey a call to action.

2. Articulates the market strategy and spells out the four goal areas necessary to achieve Operational Excellence: high satisfaction, high quality, low cost, best people (the seven KRAs were condensed into the four goal areas). Payers and patients want low-cost, hassle-free Customer service and never-fail quality.

Executive feedback. Our review panel agreed that Operational Excellence was the correct market strategy. However, there was considerable discussion about the label *low cost*. A number of suggestions were made that staff might object to *low cost* as a phrase, or that terms like *high value, cost effective,* or *best cost* might be better suited. Does the term need to be changed, or does it need to be sold?

3. Details stretch goals or BHAGs (Big Hairy Audacious Goals) for each of the four strategy elements. When management fails to set goals, or when goals are nonchallenging, the results are invariably disappointing and off target. Management experience shows that setting BHAGs enlivens the organization, gives it direction, and challenges people to do their best. It also puts management out on a limb, but then that goes with the leadership territory, doesn't it? Figure 2.3 suggests a format and identifies the objectives and measures selected by a review panel of executives from many hospitals. An actual example from Trinity Hospital in Chicago, part of the Advocate System, is shown in Figure 2.4 which details specific goals and levels to be achieved.

Executive feedback. Nearly all of our review panel said that three years was the maximum time line to project targets because of the rapid changes in the industry. The majority opinion was that the scorecard should be updated and posted monthly, although a number said that they'd settle for quarterly if monthly wasn't feasible. Monthly posting parallels the report cycle for other activity and is the desired frequency.

4. Identifies organization-wide targets for the current year and two years following. This function lets everyone know what top management wants the organization as a whole to achieve. In setting out difficult target numbers, management turns goals into BHAGs.

Figure 2.3. Organizational Strategy and BHAGs.

Organizational Goals						

High Satisfaction

Objectives	Measures	Actual		Targets			Initiatives
		MO	YTD	1999	2000	2001	
KRA: *Customer Satisfaction*							
"Wow" service	Overall percentage "excellent" rating						
	Percentile rating against other hospitals						
Zero defections	Percentage of repeat customers						

High Quality

Objectives	Measures	Actual		Targets			Initiatives
		MO	YTD	1999	2000	2001	
KRA: *Quality*							
Zero defects	Mortality, risk adjusted* (Top 100)						
	Complications, risk adjusted* (Top 100)						
Comparative performance	Progress toward Top 100 status (percentile)						

Low Cost

Objectives	Measures	Actual		Targets			Initiatives
		MO	YTD	1999	2000	2001	
KRAs: *Productivity, Economics*							
High output/input ratios	Average length of stay* (Top 100)						
	Index outpatient revenues* (Top 100)						
Expense control	Expense per adjusted discharge* (Top 100)						

Best People

Objectives	Measures	Actual		Targets			Initiatives
		MO	YTD	1999	2000	2001	
KRAs: *People Growth, Organizational Climate, Innovation*							
Optimize people growth	Number of hours training per Associate						
"Best place to work"	Percentage of excellent overall on attitude survey						
High innovation	Number of implemented DIGs and JDIs						

*Denotes a Top 100 Hospitals measurement

Figure 2.4. Trinity Hospital 1998 BHAGs.

1998 TNT BHAGs				
High Satisfaction				
Measures	Current Period	Year-to-Date	'98 Target	'97 Baseline
Inpatient composite quality score			93	84.12
Emergency room composite quality score			93	81.12
Outpatient therapies and testing composite quality score			93	82.27
Percentage of patients willing to recommend Trinity			95%	83%
High Quality				
Measures	Current Period	Year-to-Date	'98 Target	'97 Baseline
Percentage of patients rating quality excellent			63%	53%
Percentage of Associates rating Trinity as a good place to receive care			95	90
Medicare length of stay			6 days	7.01 days
JCAHO score of 100			100	100 ('95)
Low Cost				
Measures	Current Period	Year-to-Date	'98 Target	'97 Baseline
1998 Operating income (loss)			$1 million	($3.6 million)
1998 Admissions			11,200	10,169
1998 Outpatient visits			92,000	85,498
Cost per inpatient day			$1,100	$1,235
Net revenue per FTE			$102,000	$96,268
Money saved generated from implemented ideas			$3 million	$1.5 million
Best People				
Measures	Current Period	Year-to-Date	'98 Target	'97 Baseline
Number of ideas implemented hospitalwide in 1998			3,600	2,098
Training hours completed per Associate			35	20
Percentage of Associates rating Trinity as a good place to work			95	88
Percentage of Associates rating manager positively			95	90

Used by permission of Trinity Hospital, Chicago, Illinois.

Executive feedback. The measures selected herein were based on the collective opinion of the executives we surveyed. They stressed the importance of keeping the measures few in number to ease communications with Associates. Many more measures can be monitored at the direction of executives. Questions to ask are, What is really important to keep people focused on? Can they see some connection between the measure and their daily work?

Measures may prove to be a problem. Several executives reported drawing up the items they wanted measured only to find that the information system couldn't supply that information. Said one executive, "Tons of data, no intelligence." Start with what's doable and evolve the system of measures as you go. It's better to have one simple measure per BHAG that everybody understands than to have none. (This problem also highlights how much of the current reporting system doesn't really help in running the business.)

5. Provides a vehicle for department-wide goal setting. The balanced scorecard of *organizational* goals, targets, and measures is first presented to Associates in department meetings. The group then designs a list of *departmental* objectives, measures, and initiatives that fit their work situation. In other words, given the background of what top management thinks is the overall direction and plan for goals, department staffs then come up with their own pieces of the puzzle to relate to the four goal areas. These are then posted alongside the organizational goals. They would use the same format as shown in Figure 2.3, but the heading would be Team/Individual Goals instead of Organizational Goals.

Executive feedback. Departments will not have any problem in setting departmental goals that either parallel or support organization-wide goals. Department managers should be coached through the process during the first cycle. Departmental BHAGs serve to get people organized around a central idea more exciting than just doing their jobs.

General Discussion

Most executives have been enthusiastic about the balanced scorecard. They see it as a way to communicate better with departments, get everybody focused on the strategy, and bring an achievement orientation to the organization. Some even feel that the tool may help communications with the board and, in some cases, with physicians.

When one dares, and dares greatly, there is always the risk of failure. What will you do if you fail to achieve a BHAG? Of course, fear of failure is why the fainthearted never attempt to scale the mountain. As Ross Perot said of our pioneer forbears: "The cowards never started. The weak died on the way. Only the strong survived." Still, what of the dangers of daring greatly?

Executive feedback. Leaders were relatively unconcerned about setting high goals that they couldn't reach, stating that the greater risk was in establishing BHAGs that were too modest. It is time to "suck it up," said one, and get on with the job of creating greatness. When asked whether there was a risk of competitors' getting hold of a copy, most were relatively unconcerned: "They're too dumb to react," was one blunt comment. Others said some sensitivity should be shown as to where the scorecard is posted so patients don't misunderstand.

Balanced Scorecard Benefits

A balanced scorecard provides a number of advantages:

1. Balanced management control. Looking only or primarily at financial measures is like looking only at the gas gauge on a car's dashboard. It tells you whether you have enough resources to keep driving, but it won't reveal whether the engine is overheating (quality problem), how far you've driven (productivity), or whether the kids are dying for a restaurant break (Customer satisfaction). When management makes decisions with only part of the information they need, the decisions will be in error.

2. Timeliness and totality. Think about how most managers get data now. A series of unrelated reports hit their desk at different times during the month. The budget comes on the fifth of the month, the attitude opinion survey hits every two years, the Customer satisfaction data arrive quarterly. The experienced driver wants all of the gauges reporting simultaneously, and the balanced scorecard presents management information that way. By letting the manager see the total picture, at least in terms of key indicators, she is better able to understand the totality of what's happening to the business.

3. Makes upstream-downstream flow visible. Part of the problem of looking at financial measures as a primary source for decision making is that they represent organizational outputs—they are downstream outcomes of all the prior inputs and processes. For example, if innovation is low in terms of new ideas and volume of adaptive change, or if morale is falling, these souring business drivers may not affect the bottom line for a year or more. If management sees a fall-off in these indicators early on, corrective action can be taken that will save financial results a year down the time line.

4. Gives strategic direction of the enterprise. The balanced scorecard shifts thinking from a control orientation to a strategic perspective. The question in measurement shouldn't just be how much did we make or spend (though those are still good questions to ask), but rather, are we achieving our business objectives? Strategy and vision must be at the center of organizational thought, not simply control. Measuring what we want to do for Customers, what we must do in quality of services, and how people growth must accelerate provides a sense of direction often missing in the workplace. Management must not walk the treadmill but always answer the ancient question—*Quo vadis?* Where are we going? Without this sense of perspective, the organization's very future is at risk.

5. Communicates the vision and links it to operations. The balanced scorecard helps solve the problem of disconnectedness that plagues health care today. The strategic plan that executives labor over is often not even seen by managers and certainly not understood by workers. Departments function unto themselves with no sense of how their activity interconnects or relates to the work of others. By linking departmental and individual objectives to the organization's goals, the scorecard creates a greater sense of an army marching in the same direction.

6. Connects business plan strategy with work initiatives. Health care organizations are struggling to adapt to new external realities. The balanced scorecard is consistent and supportive of initiatives such as patient-focused care, quality improvement, organization redesign, cross training, and efforts to improve Customer satisfaction. Referencing both strategic direction and outcome numbers makes it easier to show why change is needed and to recognize when change efforts succeed. The rule is: Measure, make changes, measure again, then adjust the changes.

7. Provides feedback for learning. When the organization, department, or individual learns what has worked and what hasn't, it becomes possible to rethink how things should be done. This is as true for an entire organization as it is for a problem performer who receives the "shape up or ship out" talk from a supervisor. But key to any successful turnaround, or continued positive progress, is knowing where we are on the journey.

Putting the Scorecard into Action

The balanced scorecard can be a starting platform on which other initiatives can be built. Without it, the organization has nothing to shoot at. Without it, we won't know whether we hit the target.

Recommendations for Tool Installation

• Assign responsibility to a top level group. Study the concept and work out details. Be sure to get middle management input, but accountability remains with top leaders due to the impact scope.

• Boil down the philosophy. Create the organization direction summary sheet from existing vision and mission statements. Make the language short and challenging.

• Reach agreement about market strategy and goal labels. Is there agreement to pursue Operational Excellence? Are the BHAG labels acceptable?

• Set organizational measures, targets, initiatives. Look at the measures and determine which will work best for you. Because the concept is to achieve Operational Excellence, measures and targets should be tough. A number of field executives opted to shoot for at least some of the Top 100 Hospitals list of measures as a way to galvanize their organizations into action, and five of those eight measures made our final list. ("The Top 100 Hospitals" is published annually in *Modern Healthcare.* See Chapter 4 for a fuller discussion.) To win Top 100, all eight measures must be satisfied, but some measures may not be useful or appropriate to your organization's direction. Similarly, a number of new American Hospital leaders, in their atypically aggressive approach, have decided to use outside Customer measurement services as a way to get a comparative rating with other hospitals (internal measures are considered too weak, easy to hide behind.)[1] Some success has been reported with Press-Ganey. Don't get lost in the thicket over which standards to use, however. Be aggressive, not minimalist. As one executive stated, "JCAHO standards are obsolete and you'll lose your business if that's the level you produce." I wish we had at hand something better than standards of comparison sold by commercial vendors, but largely we do not. Point: Use the toughest measures and standards you can find as the safest course to pursue.

• Set outsize BHAGs. Setting stretch goals calls for courage. Managements that set lukewarm, easy-to-attain goals get little for their efforts. We must "boldly go where no person has gone before!" Here is where the risk of bogging down must be avoided. Don't let the targets become overly controlled by reductionist logic. As one leader put it: "Some targets by their nature have to be WAGs (wild-ass guesses)." Said more tastefully: These are your dreams, so dream big. If necessary, implement a shortened list of measures and targets that are easy to achieve in the interim. Don't wait to retool the whole measurement system, or slow things down in a foolish pursuit of the perfect measuring device. If necessary, go with only one target for each of the four goal areas. In this way, departments can get started rapidly to create their own objectives, measures, targets, and initiatives. A revised or expanded list of organization-wide measures and targets can be implemented in a few months. Remember, management is an action game, not an academic debate. The sooner you get something up and running, the sooner you'll see business value.

• List initiatives. These usually come from the strategic plan and are the major efforts under way in the current year, though some may be an ongoing project for several years. You will find

---

[1] See Jones and Sasser (1995) and Reichheld (1996) on the fallacies underlying Customer measurement. Among other conclusions, hospitals need to focus only on the percentage of Customers rating the organization as excellent (above average ratings don't matter because those Customers are not retention candidates), and the bad news that most hospitals are poorly rated compared to business benchmark organizations such as Disney or Marriott.

that most strategic initiatives can be neatly slotted under one of the four goal areas. Initiatives do not have to correspond directly to a measure.

• Set departmental measures, targets, initiatives. Hold departmental orientation meetings and get groups started. We suggest that managers champion a pilot effort in a few departments to get the kinks out. Another element that can aid the process is to add graphing of some measures to increase impact. The goal is to keep people focused on major outcomes, not on statistics that lose sight of the goal. Explain the organization's direction and discuss why these are important.

• Involve each department. Get departments to create measures and targets on essential elements of their operation. In some cases elements of the existing measurement system can be used, in some others they may have to be devised. Then get the groups to create a list of major initiatives the department will undertake. Don't list every little improvement, though many small actions may be feeding into the larger initiative arena.

• Convert feedback on measures into organizational and departmental action. Inevitably, measures will show that your organization has a long way to go. When people in the departments see the goals, the next item of discussion should be how to get there. A number of meetings should be held, and the group process should be allowed to provide the answers. The resulting work list of initiatives will be assigned to individuals or project teams. Past efforts to improve operations were often heroically pursued but lacked goal directedness. We anticipate that if managers use the tool correctly it will give not only direction but also motivation. The measurements will give feedback and impetus. And work initiatives will focus on adding business value.

• Celebrate the achievement of major departmental and organizational goals. Recognition and reward really add fun to all of this.

Raising standards in American health care begins with motivating the entire organization to meet high goals, the "impossible" targets that excellent people love to drag into the realm of the possible. When John Kennedy announced that the United States would go to the moon, a journey that mankind had dreamed about for thousands of years, people were astonished. Even some of the people at NASA thought the young president was reaching beyond what science would allow. Even those who had worked with the technology for years and were close to the action were taken aback by his audacious vision. On top of everything else, he wanted to do it within just ten years. Many reported spending a sleepless night that night. How could it be done? Where would one start? By the next morning, a major shift in thinking had occurred as people went to work at NASA to make the dream real.

Getting people to mobilize from a dream state to action requires BHAGs relevant to desired business outcomes, some measures, and drop-dead dates. It is the work of leadership to chart this bold course. Health care leaders can no longer journey into the future without a map if they are to discover a new and wonderful world.

Conclusion

This chapter has provided a look at strategic market positioning to assure that market requirements are met and has introduced the balanced scorecard. The scorecard is a tool that specifies the direction that Operational Excellence should take in terms of goals and the measures that determine whether progress is being made. This essential guidance mechanism also ensures that the work is focused on the identified targets. Our next chapter will deal with *strategic standardization*. It will show how an approach to standards already at work in American business can have dramatically positive results for health care organizations.

Work-Out Session

1. Would your organization benefit by specifying more precisely what it's trying to do in terms of positioning relative to its market? One approach would be to assemble a short-term task force to decide whether something like Operational Excellence with its four goals of high satisfaction, high quality, low cost, and best people makes sense.

2. How could all members of staff be given the opportunity to memorize these four goal labels?
3. What would BHAG goals do to morale and vision within your organization? Discuss the impacts that you can foresee.
4. How would departmental stretch goals affect a work team? What positive or negative factors would follow a call for them?
5. How will you measure progress toward goals? If necessary, start with an interim or partial list of measures.

Part Two

Redefining American Health Care Standards

*All men dream: but not equally. Those who dream by
night in the dusty recesses of their minds wake in the day
to find that it was vanity: but the dreamers of the day are
dangerous men, for they may act their dream with open
eyes, to make it possible.*
—T. E. LAWRENCE

The power within America's caregivers has never been more
needed or more able. The message of the market is to achieve better levels of health care performance. That certainly is the intent
of health care leaders. But how to do it?

Raising the ever-evolving health care standards within our organizations is a first step. Use of strategic standardization will continue to elevate what we do and how we do it. Reducing variability
in work processes and philosophies can also be a spur to progress.
There are many sources of standards, and the time to challenge
the idea that simple accreditation equates to excellence has come.
New ways of moving organizations forward must be found. We
must realize that *the only way to be first is first to be best.*

All of this is the natural outgrowth of Operational Excellence
and the setting of stretch goals. How good do we want to be? Can
we clear the bar if it is raised? The uncertainty of our answers is
being replaced with a new vision of a greatness we could achieve.
It is time to let our light fully shine.

Chapter Three

Winning with Strategic Standardization

A census taker called on an octogenarian Ozarkian. "Say, old timer, when's your birthday?" "Well, young feller, it's March 8." "What year?" asked the census taker. "Every year," was the answer. In life, as in organizational management, it just makes sense to standardize some things.

This chapter explores the emerging world of strategic standardization, an exciting set of concepts and approaches that translates the Operational Excellence strategy into a set of internal management practices. Strategic standardization achieves higher standards of performance, provides competitive advantage, and allows true system building to take place. It has had a tremendous impact in American business and promises to help remake the health care industry.

If you are to succeed in an increasingly competitive and cost-constrained environment you must standardize all aspects of your organization. It is a must-do strategy. If your responsibility is within a single health care organization, standardization means you must upgrade what your shop does and achieve best practices on all tasks that are worth doing. Of this you can be certain: If it isn't the best, you're just going to be somebody's lunch. Like an Alabama friend said, "If you can't run with the big dogs, stay on the porch."

If you're a leader responsible for multiple departments in different settings, or an executive looking at a multi-unit system, standardization means achieving best practices plus reducing unit variation so that units run similarly. A laissez-faire approach that allows individuals within the system to do as they please translates to high costs and loss of organizational viability.

What Standardization Is and Is Not

Let's clarify terms so that we can be certain about the actions that these terms describe. This is particularly important since they will cause important debates, and because the business promise they represent is so great.

What Is a Standard?

A *standard* is any person, model, practice, or object that becomes the frame of reference by which quality, excellence, or correctness is judged or compared. (For example, "It's the Cadillac of food processors.") It can be issued or approved by authoritative sources (for example, the American Medical Association) or emerge by general consent as best of class (Toyota overtook Taurus as best-selling automobile in America in 1997).

Standards imply a level of performance. A standard becomes the *norm* when it is regarded as typical. A standard becomes *world class* when it is ranked among the foremost in the world and is of the highest order. A *benchmark* is a standard by which something can be measured or judged. This book argues that the *norm* of American hospital performance does not represent a true *benchmark* (a higher level performance than the norm), nor does it approach *world class*.

Standards also reflect *professionalism, ethics,* and *idealism.* Work is judged to be *professional* when it is correctly done and follows approved methods. To be a professional implies a certain status and level of character. Behavioral standards are *ethical* when they support honor, personal integrity, or professional standards and ethics. At some ultimate level, standards represent our *ideals,* a sometimes unattainable standard of perfection.

Standards can be used as *measures.* Something either meets a standard or doesn't. A *yardstick* is a test used in measurement or for purposes of comparison. We are said to *gauge* something when we fix or set a standard, or try to standardize or make uniform. To *accredit* is to supply a person or organization with a credential to attest and approve that entity as meeting a prescribed standard.

Accrediting does not guarantee, it's simply one source saying that a standard has been met.

Perhaps the meanings become more powerful when we look at what it means to fail to meet standards. To *not meet standards* is to be "deviant or variant, unprofessional, amateurish, imperfect, faulty, underachieving, mediocre or average, inadequate and insufficient" (*American Heritage Dictionary,* 1992). No one in health care wants to fail meeting standards.

Among management professionals there is only one standard, and that's excellence, world class, best of breed. Why? Because management is about winning. Mediocrity is second place and second rate. Excellence is a train that runs over its competition.

Have you ever seen a dead hospital? I saw one recently. It was night and all the lights were out except for a few left on for the security detail keeping watch. Where once many lives were saved and people restored to health there was now only silence. The many hundreds of staff who had given their work lives no longer found employment here; they'd moved on to other places where leaders made better decisions. My friend explained that the organization had failed, not because of an absence of market need, but because the right decisions had not been made.

No standards, no success. No excellent organization ever filed for bankruptcy. In plain management talk, "good enough" isn't good enough when it's your child or spouse whose life is on the line. "Good enough" isn't a safe level when organization survival is at stake. After all is said and done, individuals and organizations are known by the standards they keep.

Exhibit 3.1 shows how standards have altered and elevated the course of history. As health care leaders set new standards in place, they will change the direction of our age.

Standards as Levels of Performance

If we convert these definitions of standards into a tool for management, they can be viewed as levels of performance (See Figure 3.1):

- Acceptable quality level (AQL)—These are current minimum standards or requirements. JCAHO accreditation represents this level. But current AQL standards in health care are too

Exhibit 3.1. Standards Through Time.

1403   The doge of Venice imposes world's first quarantine as a safe-guard against the Black Death. The waiting time to enter the city is standardized at forty days in 1485.

1546   The Nuremberg pharmacopoeia, published in Germany, is the first work designating the properties, actions, uses, and dosages of drugs.

1783   Noah Webster standardizes American word usage and makes spelling and pronunciation more uniform. *Webster's Spelling Book* sells more than 65 million copies in the next thirty-four years.

1798   Eli Whitney produces the first firearms with standardized, interchangeable parts.

1846   Britain adopts a standard gauge for railroads in a move that spurs development of the nation's rail system and economy.

1853   Levi Strauss can't get denim material to dye to the same shades in light colors and orders a deep indigo blue that assures him of a standard color for "blue jeans."

1858   London physician Henry Gray's *Anatomy of the Human Body* is published. The book will be a standard text for more than a century.

1869   Harvard's President Charles Eliot wins a fight with the Medical School and requires that students be given written examinations, thus elevating medical educational standards.

1879   Parke, Davis & Co. introduces liquid Ergotae Purificatus and assures physicians that dosages will be of the exact strength specified, thereby pioneering standardization of pharmaceutical drugs by chemical assay.

1901   Britain establishes statutory standards for milk to protect consumers, but pasteurization is not required, meaning that British milk remains a source of diseases.

1906   U.S. drug standards are established when the United States Pharmacopoeia and the National Formulary are recognized by the federal government.

1908   Henry Ford sells over 15 million Model T's (62 percent of all U.S. cars) before it is discontinued in 1928. The inexpensive standardized car makes Ford the largest automobile producer in the world.

Exhibit 3.1. (*continued*)

1911	The Society of Automotive Engineers publishes its first handbook, which standardizes spark plugs. The SAE goes on to standardize screw threads, bolts, nuts, and all other automotive components.
1912	The fourth down is added to U.S. football, a touchdown is given a value of six points, and the football field is standardized at 360 feet by 160 feet.
1920	Botulism from commercially canned food strikes thirty-six Americans, twenty-three die, and the U.S. canning industry, facing falling sales, imposes new production safety standards.
1921	A federal Highway Act begins to coordinate state highways and to standardize U.S. road-building practice.
1973	Nutrition-labeling regulations promulgated by the Food and Drug Administration standardize the type of information to be presented on U.S. food packages.

low and represent both a business and health threat; indeed, present definitions of what is acceptable quality are unacceptable. Managing in the fast-moving fields of medicine and health care requires a rapid, aggressive, and continuous ratcheting up of standards. Don't settle or be comfortable with this level. Getting a JCAHO score of 100 should be considered a given, a "so-what" standard.

• Benchmark levels within the industry—This is the current state of the art in terms of best results obtained by any practitioner or organization. World-class organizations seek to attain this level for competitive advantage. A problem arises when the benchmark level in one industry is lower than that in other industries; for example, the best-rated hospitals in terms of Customer satisfaction are at lower levels than benchmarks set by Disney and other leading organizations. If one settles for being the best of the mediocre, of course it is possible to be a star—but in the minor leagues. The current industry benchmarks for best practice should become the new AQL minimum standard and used as an immediate goal. We already know how to do things better in some health care

Figure 3.1. Setting Standards: What is Doable and Sensible?

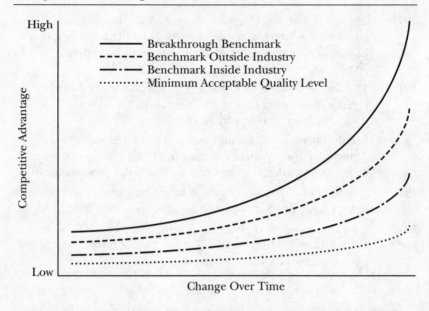

organizations than they are being done in the rest of the industry. Let's standardize on practices used in the industry's benchmark organizations and view that as the new performance floor.

• Benchmark levels outside the industry—Better-managed health care organizations are not thinking about being as good as the best hospitals. They are in hot pursuit of Lexus, Microsoft, and other approaches to management that are defining the age. Winners pursue benchmarks outside their own industry. (From a purist standpoint, benchmarks are direct comparisons between work processes in the same industry, but from a management viewpoint we want to know who's got the best idea out there regardless of industry, and then go to work to adapt it.) What does it say that hospitals visit Disney to learn Customer service from an entertainment company, but that Disney doesn't benchmark hospitals? This tougher level of performance should be a longer term goal for health care.

- Breakthrough benchmark level—This represents not simply matching the current benchmark but being innovative and daring enough to rethink how things are done and to "boldly go where no one has gone before." In each age there are leaders who do this. They are the ones who create the future.

What Is Standardization?

Once an organization has decided what level of performance to achieve, standardization can prove helpful. To *standardize* means to make things of an established size, quality, practice, or the like. It involves choosing or establishing a standard, then creating things that match it. To standardize is to *regularize*, to bring order into things, straighten things out. Another level of standardizing pushes us to the production of *uniformity*, which is to abolish differentials, equalize, normalize, or to conform to some desirable standard. A related term is *module*, which is a standardized, often interchangeable, component of a system or construction designed for easy assembly or flexible use.

Standardized means meeting or measuring up to a standard. It could mean doing things only one way (uniformity)—the best way, one hopes—or performing within a limited range of acceptably good options (regularity). For example, there may be numerous ways to handle admitting procedures, perhaps three represent the most accurate and time-efficient ways, each more appropriate to a large, medium, or small hospital. The goal of standardization would be to move toward one of these three highly satisfactory approaches.

What Standardization Is Not

Emerson said, "A foolish consistency is the hobgoblin of little minds" (Emerson, [1841] 1993). Overstandardization, standardization on nonessential tasks, or standardization on the wrong tasks is not only foolish but a waste of time, money, and effort and a choke on creativity. And standardizing mediocrity would be a disaster, an approach commonly seen in many high-control bureaucracies.

However, a *wise consistency* pushes our organizations into alignment with the best benchmarks we have. Standardization becomes not only a quest to achieve best practices, but a rejection of practices that no longer represent our best. Standardization is a death and rebirth process: "Out with the old, in with the new." Given that best practices are continually evolving, standardizing means that an onward-and-upward philosophy must underlie any organizational effort toward the imposition of a new order. It requires a constant openness at the same time that it locks in new minimums—an upward leveraging as the organization meets new benchmark levels. But remember: Always remain open to new ways of doing things or else a new rigidity enters the system.

Too much openness, however, can lead to a permissiveness that allows anybody to do anything. Under the name of "autonomy" executives can create organizations in chaos. It is an age-old governing problem: How much control should I impose, how much autonomy can I allow? The Advocate System in Chicago wisely allowed each of its facility presidents to pursue their own approach and program to Customer satisfaction and then compared outcomes. A good model first incorporates a period of openness and experimentation, then measures, and finally locks down on best practices and insists that all units comply. Once organizational elements meet the new standard, the quest for improved performance levels begins anew.

As soon as a multi-unit system has decided on its definition of standardized practices, it must allow a *skunkworks* operation to go outside the system to keep experimentation going. The term *skunkworks* was named for Kelly Johnson's freewheeling, do-anything development unit at Lockheed. Begun in 1943, it produced the first military jets. In management, the term has become synonymous with development units that are freed from all organizational constraints that make breakthrough developments impossible. Such groups are essential to engender radical and new thinking within organizations.

There are two organizational candidates to handle skunkworks assignments: Give the assignment to the best-performing unit in the system or the worst performing unit in the system. Transfer into the troubled unit some "high promotables," managers who represent the best in the talent pool, with full freedom to make massive change with the challenge to create the best unit in the system in twelve months. This one-year turnaround model has long worked successfully for Wal-Mart. The organization learns to play best-practices leapfrog, and uses natural competitive energy and prizes to drive it. Best practice does not include shutting the door on experimentation or on the evolution of better practices.

What Makes Standardization Strategic?

American business is turning increasingly to an emerging management discipline known as *strategic standardization*. There is little doubt that hospitals will embrace it in the coming decade. Brilliant hospitals will begin to use it now as part of their armament to meet business objectives and to win in the marketplace.

Strategic standardization has been shown to have a number of impacts in national and worldwide markets. It can greatly increase profitability, ensure corporate survivability, increase sales and market share, and open whole new markets. Under this view, standardization is not just a technical topic, but also a critical business issue that gives an organization a competitive edge. Many corporations have actually set up offices of strategic standardization as part of their organizational structure, including Ford, Ameritech, and Polaroid ("Competing Through Standardization," *Business Week,* 1995).[1]

An example of standardization used strategically is Bill Gates's establishment of MS-DOS (Microsoft Digital Operating System) as the computer operating system of choice. When IBM, who had commissioned the software, allowed Gates to sell it elsewhere, the rise of Microsoft to industry dominance was assured. MS-DOS can be thought of as a voluntary standards process in the private sector. No one mandated its use, but computer makers simply found that it made sense to make their machines "IBM compatible."

---

[1] My thanks to *Business Week* for publishing this special supplement. Because this is still an emerging concept, there is little written on it directly, and Internet searches came up disappointingly empty. This book would not have been written were it not for that initial inspiration.

Most standards are generated in the private sector and are followed on a voluntary basis simply because they are the best around. Microsoft is smart enough to know that once you become the standard setter, you have to raise the bar, hence the introduction of Windows 98. Make yourself obsolete with higher standards —don't let your competitor do it.

By way of contrast, Apple's operating system for computers (Mac OS), conceded for years to be both technically superior and more user friendly than MS-DOS, OS-2, and Windows 98, remains only a niche product. Apple was late to license other computer makers to use their system, and later even withdrew it from other makers. This strategic error over standards forever closed off any possibility of becoming the dominant industry player. Even if you have the better mouse trap, the world won't use it if it is not easily accessible.

A clear example of how standards can dominate is the U.S. Pharmacopoeia (USP), an independent scientific organization that establishes legally recognized quality standards for the use of medicines. USP standards are recognized as official and are enforced by the Food and Drug Administration (FDA). The combination of the USP standards with FDA backing has made USP standards de facto world standards. Indeed, most countries around the world do not have the equivalent of a USP or FDA. In many nations, health regulations simply require that medicines used in their country have FDA approval (USP standards).

The U.S. federal government is the largest creator and user of standards, some 52,000 of them. There are 43,000 standards in the American private sector, for a total of 95,000 written documents specifying, for example, the best roofing materials, allowable contaminants per million parts of water, or pounds of load in building trusses. There is an even larger number of de facto industry standards that are basically determined by widespread acceptance in the free market. Some de facto standards that are accepted as best of breed include Heinz ketchup, Libby's pumpkin pie mix, French's mustard, Kleenex, even Elvis. De facto standards are accepted by the market majority, or important segments of it, but not necessarily by everyone.

What are the largely de facto standards in health care? Most are not regulated or issued by others, and most are different for the various functions within the organization. That is, de facto standards exist both in clinical and nonclinical aspects of the organization; they are the ways in which individuals think things should be done. Another way to think of them would be as professional, technical, or managerial standards; as human or machine performance standards; or as standards of time or quality for particular work processes. Each department needs to identify an organizing scheme that will define standards appropriate to its work—don't just let people do things "any old which way." There should also be some housewide standards, such as greeting patients by name or answering phones by the third ring. Define and organize standards any way that works, get them published, and involve people through training and problem solving to achieve the levels of performance to which all are committed. The goal is to become the de facto standard in the community, state, or region for excellence in care.

There are famous examples of companies failing to establish a new de facto standard: Sony's Betamax was unable to replace the existing industry VHS standard. Customers, acknowledging Betamax's superiority, just didn't think the value was worth the cost and inconvenience of changing. But the same electronics market was willing to forsake 8-track for cassette tapes, and cassettes for CDs. And what about the less than brilliant decision to offer New Coke and abandon Classic Coke? The market immediately forced reinstatement of America's most desired soft drink standard. The market, individual Customers, favors *higher standards* in products and services, but only if they are also *worth the cost.*

Japanese automakers overwhelmed Detroit in the 1970s with cars that met higher quality and performance standards than anything being made in the United States. This private sector standard was quickly accepted by American consumers. Detroit automakers had no choice but make cars "as good as the Japanese" —the standards had been redefined.

Could a similar, strategically important first strike be made by an American health care system against its competitors? The use of strategic standardization could be particularly beneficial for health providers who propose early on that their standards be accepted for national use. Consider just this example in the press recently: "Health care reform is one example where the U.S.

is poised for significant government regulatory and procurement changes. There is bipartisan and unanimous support in the area of health care administration, including the need to reduce and simplify paperwork. The development of standards related to computer-based patient records is one key component" ("Competing Through Standardization, *Business Week,* 1995).

What Leaders Say About Strategic Standardization

How do leaders in other competitive industries see the strategic nature of the standards issue? Many corporations have established offices of strategic standardization, and there are now corporate titles such as vice president of standardization. The view seems to be emerging that standardization is truly strategic and vital to business interests, and that it leads to competitive advantage. Executive proponents of strategic standardization don't believe that following standards set by others (as in JCAHO accreditation) is an approach leading to success. The organization that sets the standard is the leader.

William Hudson, CEO of AMP, Inc., states: "Companies taking an aggressive approach to standards can derive critical advantage in shorter time-to-market and a higher 'hit' ratio, while those adopting a defensive posture of simply creating products that conform to existing standards risk falling behind the learning curve" ("Competing Through Standardization," *Business Week,* 1995). If an organization is focused on simply conforming to existing JCAHO standards, would it risk falling behind a competitor who is in hot pursuit of becoming the industry benchmark? Would that competitor, in aggressively copying best practices, be moving ahead and up the learning curve?

Michael Gorman of Ameritech declares in *Business Week* ("Competing Through Standardization," 1995): "We've moved from viewing standards as a technical concern to seeing them as a basic Customer and marketing issue. If we can involve end users in standards development . . . we can increase American competitive advantage." Would a hospital that involved its patients and physicians in setting new standards and then pursued those issues important to end users increase its competitive advantage? If your health care provider listened to you intently, then altered service elements to meet your needs, would it make a difference to you and your family?

Is there some inevitability to standardization? Is this an idea whose time has come? It now appears that organizations that do not move upward in their standards and who do not move to standardize processes will be left behind. Alex Trotman of Ford Motor Company states: "There are only two kinds of organizations: Those that have embraced a standards process, and those that will" ("Competing Through Standardization," *Business Week*, 1995).

George Fisher, CEO of Kodak and chairman of U.S. Council of Competitiveness, says, "As we look to the future, standards will become even more important. American companies must understand that standardization is a strategic business issue that has a direct impact on new product development. There is a direct relationship between leadership in standards and leadership in technology. American standard bodies must lead the way in international activities" ("Competing Through Standardization," *Business Week*, 1995). Based on the experience at hand in the corporate world, is it reasonable to conclude that there is a direct link between standards leadership in health care and leadership in the development of better health care services? Raising standards, which is a lot of work, produces better and newer services, which leads to competitive advantage and profitability as the following case study demonstrates.

Standardization at Marriott

Marriott is the world's largest and most successful hotel chain. With nearly 2,000 facilities under its flag (primarily managed, not owned), the Marriott standardized approach produces a dependable and pleasing "Honored Guest" (Customer) experience. Marriott neatly solved the diversification trap by selling off food services and other unrelated businesses to partners, and by segmenting the market's price points into Fairfield Inns, Marriott Courtyards, Marriott Hotels, Marriott Suites, Marriott Resorts, and Four Seasons. Although each segment runs under separate, autonomous managements, each is governed by standardized culture, reporting systems, technology, suppliers, and, most important, a people-selection and training system that produces the key feature of what the Customer encounters—a helpful person.

The standardization strategy, begun under the demanding founder, Willard Marriott, was extensively driven deep into the organization by his son Bill. His commonsense advice has clear applications for American health care (Marriott and Brown, 1997):

We are sometimes teased about our passion for the Marriott Way of doing things. If you happen to work in the hospitality industry, you might already be familiar with our encylopedic procedural manuals, which include what is probably the most infamous of the bunch: a guide setting out sixty-six separate steps for cleaning a hotel room in less than half an hour.

Maybe we *are* a little fanatical about the way things should be done. But for us, the idea of having systems and procedures for everything is very natural and logical: If you want to produce a consistent result, you need to figure out how to do it, write it down, practice it, and keep improving it until there's nothing left to improve. (Of course, we at Marriott believe that there's *always* something to improve.)

Why do we feel that doing things consistently is so important? The simple answer is that it's the solid foundation upon which virtually every aspect of Marriott rests. If we've got our systems down cold, everything else becomes much easier.

Think about it for a moment. At the most basic level, systems help bring order to the natural messiness of human enterprise. Give 100 people the same task—without providing ground rules— and you'll end up with at least a dozen, if not 100, different ways of doing it. Try that same experiment with a few thousand people, and you end up with chaos. Efficient systems and clear rules help everyone to deliver a consistent product and service. . . .

One of our chief aims is to provide our customers with service free of hassles and surprises. Road-tested systems and SOPs make this possible by taking the element of surprise out of situations where surprise is the last thing a guest wants. We try to provide a level of service so dependable that a guest can land on our doorstep virtually asleep on her feet and not miss a "zzz" while we register and usher her to a room for the night.

That level of consistency gives customers confidence in your brand name and incentive to come back again and again. We could not have expanded as quickly, widely, or profitably as we have over the years if we had to reinvent the wheel every time we unveiled a new hotel, resort, restaurant, or senior living community. Or if we were forced to reintroduce ourselves to the world each time a new facility opened. . . .

Systems have been deeply ingrained for so long in our corporate culture that I'm always a little surprised when I come across companies that aren't as devoted to them as we are. Among our peers in the hospitality industry, I often see wasted opportunities to improve performance, simply because no one seems to be focusing on developing, much less implementing and maintaining, systems and standards. The result is uneven, unreliable, and often unremarkable service. . . .

In Marriott's case, our principal product is probably not what you think it is. . . . Yes, we "sell" room nights, food and beverage, and time-shares. But what we're really selling is our expertise in managing the processes that make those sales possible. And that expertise rests firmly on our mastery of thousands of tiny operational details.

It is the mastery of thousands of operational details that health care is now beginning to pursue and combine into the standardized, high-performance delivery system of tomorrow.

Dealing with New Business Realities

Standardization will prevail in American health care precisely because it responds to the new reality of having to produce flawless service outcomes at ever lower cost. Whether the terminology is managed care, capitation, covered lives, HMO, or contracting, it all means the same thing: Resources are and will remain constrained. Other forecasts are that litigation by angry Customers will increase if the system does not change, and that employers will select providers almost exclusively from outcomes measures. These realities will have to be managed aggressively to win the game in the coming era. The best answer is standardized best practices applied everywhere in the health care system.

Core Competencies for Cost Control

The new era of standardization is driven by the need for the organization to achieve core competencies that meet the requirements of the market. By being really good at these things, health care organizations will thrive. Based on trend data and the thinking of futurists, here are some elements that have to be mastered in the near term. Use them as a checklist for what needs to be done in your shop.

Satisfy contractor requirements. Increasingly, hospitals will find that they are in the contracting business. Dealing with mass purchasers, which necessitates specifying inputs and outputs, will require that an organization runs standardized systems that can produce care with little variation in costs, services, and time. It's doubtful that a nonstandardized system can meet contracted requirements. Although health care may not be an assembly line business, borrowing some assembly line techniques may be possible to reduce the variance in the pieces that are not strictly mechanical.

Integration of doctors. As prescribers, physicians control 62.5 percent of patient care costs (Kaiser Permanente, 1994). Physician integration translates to capture, control, and credentialing.

- Capture: Most organizations are now well along in recruiting and tying into their referral patterns the physicians, general practitioners, and internists, especially, who can feed the system that patients need, offering whatever benefits, practice support, or ownership options that are available.
- Control: This includes adjusting the mix of general practitioners versus specialists, requiring that their practice not be split with other hospitals, doing whatever is necessary to be their hospital of choice, and moving physicians to standardization of clinical protocols and supply and technology usage.
- Credentialing: NCQA accreditation requires that an HMO's physicians be currently licensed, up to speed with continuing education, and free from legal or otherwise problematic histories. Utilization review and quality assurance are also part of the equation. Economic credentialing means that doctors whose approach to practice costs significantly more than their peers may not be invited to practice.

Patient-centered care. As one way to start moving away from a departmentalized, vertical organization to a more horizontal work flow, patient-centered care will produce faster throughput, better quality, and lower cost. In essence, the organization's work processes must be retrofitted to the Customer, rather than asking the Customer to fit into the "way we do things here." Under this heading should be included any reengineering, restructuring, or organizational renewal strategy that gets to the same general end of more efficient throughput.

Pursuit of operational efficiency. Hospitals are notoriously inefficient because of the high variance in the number and type of outputs they try to provide and the range of inputs they permit. Many suppliers mean more management problems to contend with, and higher per unit costs of supplies ordered. Fewer suppliers mean just the opposite. So the prescription for *lean* in the "lean, mean machine" requires going on a diet: fewer inputs, fewer services offered, and fewer outputs. But for what comes into, is processed, and then produced, there will be a much greater intensity of focus to do each step flawlessly and quickly. Speed and accuracy are the outputs needed to win. A sloppy system is a non sequitur: If it's sloppy, it isn't a system.

Standardized practices. Malpractice, whether medical or managerial, occurs when a practitioner does not follow the known truths of his profession and practices against the grain. Letting physicians practice with procedures ten years out of date is an area that will have to be addressed. Once we know the best practice, why would we want to do it any other way? Hospitals will need to standardize clinical processes into a set of standard protocols followed by all. With computerized expert systems already available, it would be foolish not to have computer validation of diagnoses, a second opinion from an expert system database. On occasion, this will mean that physicians will be presented with data suggesting that the course of action they're considering is contraindicated.

Information management. What is needed is a seamless web of real-time data connecting all users in the hospital, outlying clinics, physicians' offices, and pharmacies. Computerized systems can by default require standardized performance from the humans who use them. Software controls that won't permit entering an adult dosage when the patient record indicates this is a child, or that won't permit moving to the next screen if some vital piece of information hasn't been entered, produce something closer to flawless performance. Although this project is well along in some places, a wide discrepancy remains in other locations. The Customer, accustomed to computer-managed information in other walks of life, is often amazed when departments fifty feet down the hall from each other are unable to relay who the patient's doctor is or track the Customer's phone number. Health care is an applied science—if you can't figure out the technology, don't play in the game.

The attainment of these core competencies requires standardization. There is no other way. I was confronted with this brave new world when filling a prescription recently. My Walgreen's pharmacist, using such a computer database, was alerted to a drug interaction with other medicines I was already taking. Although my family doctor is excellent, why was this data and technology not available in his office, and the problem caught there?

Benefits of Standardization

The new standardized system is happening now. It is a revolution well on its way. Yet confusion and doubt about its outcomes are widely present. What are the payoffs that will be worth the work?

Common Systems, Uncommon Benefits

Standardization responds to the new business realities in a way that goes far beyond mere survival. A standardized work system based on a commonly shared culture produces a number of benefits to the organization and its stakeholders—its Customers, practitioners, and staff. Here are some benefits of a standardized work system:

Common training programs. Once best practices are in place, it is possible to have one training program for those procedures instead of multiple approaches within the same organization or across a multi-unit chain.

Makes least able staff able. Systems remove work from people and place it in machines and procedures. To expect everybody to remember everything is no longer realistic. Create a system that requires adherence rather than many people doing what they feel like. Such a system is far easier to control, and it makes it simpler for people to do their job.

Frees up superior talent. When staff members are supported by a system carrying some of the burden, they can attend to higher-order tasks. In management, *problems* are usually associated with things we designed and decided yesterday and that are going wrong in the present. *Opportunities* are associated with the future. Systems free up talent to work on opportunities rather than endlessly working to fix problems and redo work associated with nonbest practices.

Reduces development time and cost. "Plug and play" becomes doable when a best practice, already developed, can be used in another setting without having to laboriously reinvent the wheel.

Slick systems. Efficient systems always reduce operating costs and increase speed. This is the financial payoff in a managed care environment.

Ends one-by-one renewal. This benefit is particularly important for multihospital systems. Instead of treating each institution as a free-standing entity, introducing an already developed best practice standard is an easier and faster way to reduce variance between institutions. Common elements can be swapped between institutions rather than custom-fitted to each location.

Protects the Customer. Quality must mean dependable, reliable outcomes. Controlled systems lead to fewer errors and are far less inconvenient and confusing to the Customer.

Reduction of quality variation. A common account in the press on the theme of health care's nonstandardized systems is that of an organization that performs quite well for years but then commits some horror. One story shared with me by a frustrated CEO was of two patients with the same name and same birth date who were admitted on the same day. You guessed it. The one patient's surgical procedure was performed on the other. A computer scan of a patient ID number might have caught the problem. Reputation, which takes years to achieve, can be lost overnight when a nonbest practice is used.

Peak performance. Ultimately, whether a hospital is stand-alone or part of a multi-unit system, the only way to compete and to attain and sustain a competitive advantage is consistently to do a better job than the other guy.

Standardization helps to make all these outcomes a reality. The argument for best practices is clearly in favor of making the effort.

Dangers and Risks of Standardization

Even good medicine can be bad for you if not administered correctly. Be sure you don't fall into one of these traps:

Picking the wrong model. TQM is one avenue toward best practices. However, it is not a silver bullet or a panacea, nor is it appropriate for many hospitals. Rather than buying a prepackaged program, examine all the options. Combine eclectically the truths that all these approaches have. One key characteristic of a right model is that it will be open-ended rather than closed, meaning that a lot of input and control is possible by those affected by the changes.

Autocratic imposition. You can get standardization the way Mussolini did—just pull on your jackboots and start issuing orders. But remember, implementing standardization in such a way that kills the culture or causes it to lose effervescence is not what you want. As in just about everything else managerial, the *skills* in change management are what make the project succeed or fall, not the excellence of the content.

Organizational stalling. Organizations have a built-in bias to do nothing. A worst case scenario is one in which different power groups have assumed various positions and fortified their defenses. Someone is going to have to drive change. How will you increase or strengthen driving forces? How will you weaken or decrease resistant forces? Good political and leadership skills are required, not just the good logic that standardization represents.

Poor implementation. This is less a change management issue in the emotional sense and more simply a poor plan of work execution.

When I was a student, I spent some time in England. While there, I bought a tape recorder and was handed a bag full of various electrical plugs with my purchase. "What, pray tell, are these for?" I asked. Said the salesman, "We never standardized electrical wall outlets in the United Kingdom, so we've thoughtfully provided you with plugs for the ones you're most likely to encounter."

Worse yet, my apartment had outlets of three types, all different, so I had to purchase various adapters. So much wasted on account of nonstandardization!

Executive Reactions to Standardization

In a survey of health care executives, ninety-five participants at the 1996 ACHE Congress, half from single hospitals and half from multi-unit systems, were asked to respond to a number of central hypotheses regarding the value of standardization (V. C. Sherman, unpublished). There was no significant difference in response rates between the two groups, which included similar proportions of department directors, VPs, and CEOs (see Table 3.1).

This brief survey produced three primary findings:

1. The argument for standardization is largely accepted in all of its ramifications; that is, standardized best practices would elevate standards and reduce organizational variation within systems to the benefit of quality and cost.
2. Standardization is already well under way. Although the term means many things to many people, it is clear that a widespread effort to improve operations is already at work. Clinical protocols lead the parade and improved management brings up the rear; the latter is a symptomatic problem that is retarding industry progress.
3. Leaders are clearly frustrated by resistance and a slower adaptation than they would like. Much of this is traceable to variance in management practice and lack of shared strategic vision.

To verify the views of these civilian health care leaders, the author distributed a similar survey at the 1996 Department of Defense TriCare worldwide health meeting in Washington, D.C. (V. C. Sherman, unpublished). Representing approximately 200 hospitals and 500 clinics worldwide, America's military runs what may be the most complex health care system in the world. Among seventy-eight officers responding, there was marked agreement with the general arguments for standardization, substantial ongoing efforts to make best practice improvements across a broad spectrum of work processes, and frustration with resistance from

Table 3.1. Executive Reactions to Standardization.

% Yes	% No	Elements of the Standardization Argument Agreed With:
96	4	1. For quality and cost, the industry should move toward standardization of best practices
95	5	2. A low-cost/Operational Excellence market strategy is right for hospitals to pursue
93	7	3. Individual hospitals should move toward a best practices model of management
91	9	4. Raising standards ahead of rest of the industry would provide a competitive advantage
91	9	5. Multihospital systems should move toward standardization among units
87	13	6. Management of hospitals would be improved by following corporate best practices

% Yes	% No	We're Pursuing Standardization in These Areas:
92	8	1. Clinical paths and treatment protocols
85	15	2. Standardizing information systems
84	16	3. Standardizing in materials management
81	19	4. Standardizing financial procedures/forms
78	22	5. Standardizing in pharmacy
75	25	6. Standardizing human resource departmental procedures/forms
42	58	7. Standardizing management practices, e.g., MBO, meeting management

% Yes	% No	Standardization Concerns Regarding the Organization:
79	21	1. Change management is a bigger problem than change content*
59	41	2. We have too much variance in managerial philosophy to allow standardization
19	81	3. At present, our standardization efforts are timely and on schedule
19	81	4. I am concerned that standardization will mean loss of managerial freedom/autonomy
17	83	5. At present, our standardization efforts are adequate, appropriate, and sufficient
10	90	6. I am concerned that standardization gains won't be worth the effort or costs

*Human resistance is more of a problem than the items being changed top leadership to pursue standardization as an objective. As one might expect from this group, there was a strong expression to seize the high ground of setting new world benchmarks ahead of the civilian sector. *Semper fi!*

Health care leaders resonate positively with the notion of strategic standardization. What seems to be needed is a clearly articulated approach to standardization, for executives are repeatedly asking for a road map. Where should we go? How can we get there?

What Standardization Means to You

Standardization represents different goals depending on one's responsibility in health care.

For a *hospital executive,* the challenge is to achieve best practices housewide. This includes clinical and nonclinical areas. As I explain later, initially this can provide a competitive advantage against other providers. If one provider bests its competitors in this regard, continued viability in the era of managed care will be assured. Best practices always favor the three primary targets of the business: cost, quality, and Customer retention.

For the *health system leader,* the goal is twofold: to achieve best practices in each organizational entity, and to rationalize the system and reduce unit variation. If there are twenty-three hospitals in the chain, do you need twenty-three different billing procedures, information systems, and physician credentialing approaches? In continuous quality improvement (CQI) terms, there is too much variance, and too much variance inevitably leads to a system that is "out of control." Although uniform standardization may be too much to achieve in the short run, reducing the amount of variation to two or three approaches in department categories may be realistic in the short term.

For a *department manager,* the primary task is to keep up with the state of the art (best practices) in technical and management terms. Are we following the most current thinking? Does what we do measure up to the tests of quality and cost? One director of nursing noted that their nursing procedures manual was hopelessly out of date, even dangerous if followed. Her nursing council decided to adopt the *Lippincott Manual of Nursing Practice,* with its continuously revised editions, and to make sure that internal training regimes followed it. Not only was quality assisted, but think of the immense savings in time on the part of her staff who did not have to rewrite these procedures.

For a *physician,* the focus is how to keep skills and knowledge on the cutting edge as knowledge continues to explode. Though communication of new findings provides timely news of changes in clinical practice, why is radical mastectomy still widely used when research points to lumpectomy as the preferred procedure? Physicians' prescribing habits are another example of a doctor sticking with an older drug because of past good experience with it even though newer products are often more efficacious. And how much longer can hospitals order equipment and supplies that only one physician uses? Obviously, this is an area of much debate. But it is a debate that must happen, and the answers will lead to greater standardization and a lowering of risk and cost as the following case study demonstrates.

Standardization at Southwest

To help think through what standardization might mean in health care, let's look at a case in the airline industry.[2] Many of the principles that will work in health care have already succeeded at Southwest Airlines. Southwest has adopted an Operational Excellence strategy in its market positioning. Let's examine how high satisfaction, high quality, low cost, and best people combine to create one of the most remarkable success stories in American business.

By any analysis Southwest Airlines is a classic illustration of the power of contrarian thinking. It combines the rigor of standardization with a rambunctious culture. Stories of its maverick CEO, Herb Kelleher, voted the "best CEO in America" in 1994 (Labich 1994), and its freewheeling culture set it apart. Recently, Kelleher's book, *Nuts,* became a runaway best seller and a must-read for American executives.

RESULTS OF OPERATIONAL EXCELLENCE

When it comes to getting best results, Southwest excels like no other in its industry (see Figure 3.2). The airline made the transition from an expanding regional to a national carrier in 1996 when it opened service to Boston. Clearly its profit margins are directly related to its higher productivity, both in terms of planes and Customers per employee. In a number of recent years, Southwest

---

[2]This case study is largely derived from Weidner (1990) and the best practices Internet library of the Department of Labor.

Figure 3.2. Southwest Airlines Compared to Competitors.

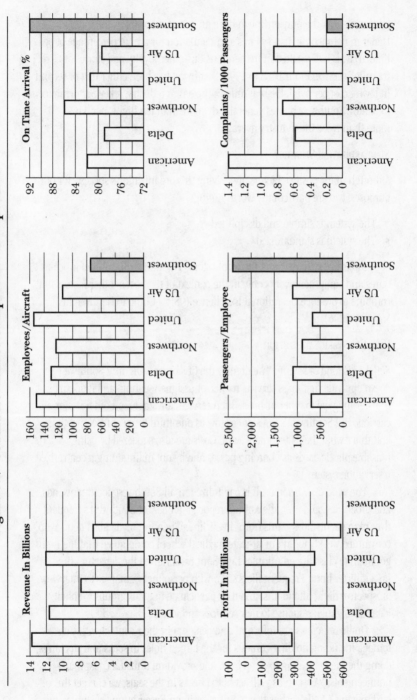

Source: Chicago Tribune.

has been either the only airline to have an operating profit or the industry leader in net income. Its low fares and reputation for a high percentage of on-time arrivals has resulted in tremendous Customer loyalty and stories of "extra mile" service. From 1988 to 1998, Southwest has been either first or second in lowest cost per available seat mile in the entire industry, a key performance indicator. Southwest planes generally fly more than ten flights per day—more than twice the industry average.

STANDARDIZATION STRATEGY

Although many positive factors are driving this organization's success, for our purposes, two are particularly worth noting:

- The system is simple and disciplined
- The system is standardized

To standardize systems is not the whole story. The standardization of procedures and equipment works only in the context of the host of other factors that combine to produce Operational Excellence ("Slow Climb to New Heights," *Success,* 1996).

HIGH CUSTOMER SATISFACTION

Kelleher is fond of saying, "We dignify the Customer." Dignify? Southwest doesn't provide first-class service, meals, or assigned seating, and it doesn't transfer luggage to other airlines. Such services are staples on other major air carriers. But Southwest's fares are as low as one-third those of its competitors, and that's what their Customers want. Costs are also squeezed by using reusable plastic cards as boarding passes and by not maintaining a centralized reservation system.

The word *Customer* itself is capitalized in all Southwest documents, ads, and brochures, and even the annual report. Members of Southwest's frequent flyer plan get birthday cards from the airline. When five medical students who commuted weekly to an out-of-state medical school complained that the flight got them to class fifteen minutes late, Southwest moved the departure time up a quarter hour. Frequent fliers sit in with personnel managers to interview prospective flight attendants, and they participate in focus groups to solicit ideas or to gauge response to new services and ideas.

On board, crews are informal and personal in their contact with Customers, including holding contests for the largest holes in socks and stockings, doing the safety briefing to a rap beat, and providing unusual cockpit announcements: "As soon as y'all set both cheeks in the seats, we can get this ol' bird moving." Kelleher has flown on Easter in an Easter bunny costume, and has dropped in at maintenance hangers at 2 A.M. dressed as "Klinger" from television's MASH. The humor has a purpose: "What's important is that a Customer should get off the airplane feeling: 'I didn't get from A to B. I had one of the most pleasant experiences I ever had and I'll be back for that reason.'"[3]

Competitors offer a package that includes meals and higher rates of lost bags and late arrivals, whereas Southwest serves only peanuts but gets you there on time, with your bags, and for cheap. Customers seem to favor the second package.

HIGH QUALITY OUTCOMES

Standardization creates a minimalist system. Simpler systems have fewer things that can go wrong. Southwest flies only the Boeing 737, whereas other carriers, like American, fly as many as twelve types of aircraft. Multiple plane varieties multiply complexity through the system: twelve cabin-attendant training programs, twelve parts inventories, twelve pilot certification and re-training schedules, ad infinitum. Standardization on one type of aircraft allows easy substitution of personnel from one flight to another. Thorough knowledge of the craft allows faster turnarounds, better inventory control, and tougher negotiating leverage with suppliers. For example, by flying only Boeing 737s, Southwest has kept costs low by stocking only one type of titanium wing nut instead of six or seven. This simple, unvarying system element gives Southwest a competitive advantage that is unmatched by any other airline. Standardization is at the core of Operational Excellence.

Contrast that with a report in the *Chicago Tribune* of what is now happening within the industry as other airlines now race to catch up in the standardization arena ("Keeping It Simple," 1994):

- For many airlines, fleets have grown into a hodgepodge of models. . . . All require their own spare parts. Crews must undergo long training sessions to learn the nuances of each plane. Southwest pilots only need to know their way around one cockpit layout.
- The mishmash has gotten so costly that airlines . . . are looking to simplify their fleets. . . . "Increasingly you'll see airlines become supplied by a single manufacturer," said [a Salomon Brothers analyst].
- That's where the savings come in. It's like having a garage full of Chevys, Fords, and Dodges and having to stock oil filters for all. But in the airline

---

[3] Quotes of Kelleher throughout this section are excerpted from Labich (1994) and "Slow Climb to New Heights" (1996).

industry parts can cost millions. And the less time $100,000-per-year pilots spend in classrooms, the more money the airline makes.

- In hindsight, the costly lessons of motley fleets seem obvious, raising the question of how the airlines got into such a predicament. One answer is that many airlines took the best deal that came along when they were ready to buy.

Getting people to understand the team concept is also a big part of Southwest's success. Each operating unit at Southwest identifies internal Customers and focuses on their needs. Mechanics target pilots who fly the planes they maintain, and marketing staffers target reservation agents. Departments shower one another with gifts, pizza, and ice cream as tokens of Customer devotion, or in appreciation for a job well done. Employees who earn repeated commendations — sometimes called Love Reports — may earn free perks: a free meal or a choice parking spot.

Quality outcomes? Southwest is the only airline that has never had a major accident — the only airline that has never killed a passenger.

LOW COST AND FINANCIAL FACTORS

The airline business is not all fun and games. Only tight control of costs makes Southwest's low fares possible. Southwest's costs, lowest by far in the airline industry, are 29 percent lower than Delta's and 32 percent lower than United's. Southwest, however, recorded a 256 percent increase in profits in 1991 and is growing at the rate of 15 percent annually. Financially conservative, Southwest was second only to Delta in financial strength in 1990. What's the secret of Southwest's contrarian success?

Southwest's approach is entirely different from that of any other airline. Southwest specializes in high-frequency, short-distance flights. All of Southwest's flights are under two hours of flight time, and many are under sixty minutes. Fares are cut-rate: when Braniff's Dallas-Houston fare was $62, Southwest's fare was just $15 (Braniff did not survive). Kelleher doesn't see other airlines as Southwest's competition: "We're pricing ourselves against Ford, GM, Chrysler, Toyota, and Nissan. The traffic is already there, but it's on the ground. We take it off the highway and put it on the airplane."

Planes are kept in the air as much as possible so that revenue per aircraft is maximized. Southwest's turnaround time to unload passengers, clean and service the plane, and board passengers is around fifteen minutes for 70 percent of its flights, and 10 percent of flights have a turnaround time of ten minutes compared to an hour averaged by most other major carriers.

When fuel costs increased rapidly due to the Iraqi invasion of Kuwait, about a third of Southwest's 8,600 employees contributed voluntarily from their pay to buy aviation fuel for the airline. Kelleher says he didn't know about the "Fuel from the Heart" program until he received a banner signed by all the employees who made the pledges. "We realized that, on the average of twice a decade, you're going to be faced with difficult times. I tell the people here that we must always manage so that we do well in bad times."

BEST PEOPLE AND CULTURE

"The people who work here don't think of Southwest as a business," Southwest Airlines CEO Herbert Kelleher says proudly. "They think of it as a crusade." This pride is especially evident at a time when air transportation is viewed by the market as a commodity, lowest fares win market share, and airlines build volume while racking up record losses. Southwest Airlines has been recognized as one of *The 100 Best Companies to Work for in America* by authors Robert Levering and Milton Moskowitz (1994). Southwest's annual turnover rate is only 3 to 4 percent, the lowest in the airline industry. Says Kelleher, "If you don't treat your own people well, they won't treat other people well."

Cooperation among Southwest's unionized workforce is high. Rather than fostering a confrontational relationship with Southwest's unions, the airline negotiated flexible work rules that improve its competitiveness. For example, flight attendants and pilots pick up the trash on the plane after a flight; cleaning crews are only used at the end of the day. Kelleher says, "Our employees have been very cooperative. They see Southwest as an ongoing institution, so they're thinking about 2010, not next Wednesday. We don't furlough anybody, so we have to be lean all the time." Whereas employees of nearly all other airlines wear uniforms, Southwest flight attendants' attire is shorts, casual shirts, and sneakers—Customers report this makes them seem more "approachable." (Hospital patient surveys report approachability to staff is greatest with housekeepers and aides, least with executives in suit and tie).

Southwest is fond of saying that they hire people with "great attitudes." Says Kelleher: "If you don't have a great attitude, we don't want you, no matter how skilled you are. We can change skill levels through training. We can't change attitude."

No, managing health care is not the same as running an airline. But we could adapt and creatively expand elements of what Southwest does as we reconceptualize how we want to design twenty-first century delivery systems: Simplify the system, improve the work climate and culture, and standardize the technology.

Conclusion

This chapter has outlined the exciting new concept of strategic standardization and pointed out that raising standards is not only the right thing to do but also provides competitive advantage. Part of raising standards is reducing variances in procedures, technology, even attitudes. This standardization produces dramatically lower costs and higher quality through greater control. In the following chapter we discuss how to define standards, what sources of standards to use, and where standards are heading. These insights will help us apply standards and standardization as tools for successful organizational evolution.

Work-Out Session

1. If you were in charge of Southwest Memorial, a fictional new health care subsidiary of Southwest Airlines, which elements of operational management would you bring forward into the hospital? Which elements of corporate culture?
2. Do you think that standardization can be a competitive strategy in health care? How would higher standards, and making sure that work processes match best practices, give your organization a competitive edge?
3. Where do the standards in your organization lack clarity? Where is your organization falling behind best practices in what it offers Customers?
4. What are the dangers of not differentiating the services of your organization? What problems arise when your Customers think of health care at your organization as a commodity, no different from that found at any other provider? What could a health care organization do that would truly be seen as different and of value to the market?
5. Should your organization redefine its relationships with Customers and Associates? Do you see these cultural variables as "nice to do" or as core to the successful implementation of Operational Excellence? Are they the outcomes or the causes of success?

Chapter Four

Existing Standards Are Not Enough

It's always easier to plan a trip than actually making the journey. Paul had planned a trip to Paris for a very long time, and the day after his retirement, he was on a plane. His old friend Herb met him at the airport on his return, and asked, "Well, Paul, how was Paris?"

"Oh, it was fine," replied the weary traveler, "but I wish I'd gone twenty years ago."

"When Paris was really Paris, eh?" asked Herb sympathetically.

"No, when Paul was really Paul."

In thinking through any journey, we always begin by defining our destination. Where do we want to go? In health care, what standards do we want to reach? And where can we look to find better standards? In this chapter we'll look at these questions through the eyes of Customers, employers, and payers, all of whom have higher expectations as shown in recent years. What old standards and destinations no longer serve very well? What newer standards can be used to help drive organization performance? We will find that some of these standards we can borrow, but some we will have to create on our own.

Is the JCAHO Failing?

Approximately 4 percent of the 33 million patients who enter the nation's hospitals each year will be injured or die because of caregiver negligence or malpractice or other problems in the health care system (Brennan and others, 1991; Leape and others, 1991).

More people will die from their health care encounters than will die from shootings and car accidents combined. The dimensions of health care as health hazard are astounding, yet no government agency, federal or state, maintains a record of this epidemic. The sites for these potentially deadly individual and isolated encounters are hospitals. *Nearly all these hospitals were accredited by the Joint Commission for the Accreditation of Health Care Organizations (JCAHO).*

Central to decisions about how high standards should be set and how best to implement and enforce them is the question of what to do with the JCAHO. Established in 1951 as an educational organization, the group was not originally intended to be a regulatory agency. It has never been entirely comfortable with that role, arguing that accreditation should be a voluntary process to achieve "beneficial effects through a combination of evaluation, education, and consultation" (Roberts, Coale, and Redman, 1987).

A 1995 study that examined injuries related to medication in two highly regarded hospitals found a rate of 1,900 injuries per hospital per year. The researchers concluded that one-third of these errors were preventable, and that many were caused by poor practices and procedures for ordering, dispensing, and administering drugs (Bates and others, 1995; Leape and others, 1991). This finding demonstrates that the system is as much at fault as human negligence. *Nearly all these hospitals were accredited by the JCAHO.*

As an accreditation service, the JCAHO sets the standards and procedures by which the public is supposed to be safeguarded. How effective has that approach been? Is it time to drastically alter or end it? Can the JCAHO effectively monitor the nation's health care organizations? Are the criticisms of it fair? The basic question is simply whether standards of care are met, and if not, what needs to be changed. This question is not about blaming the JCAHO, or other regulators, for individual errors occurring all over the country. Recently, a JCAHO surveyor, a respected former hospital CEO, said, "You should have seen things in the old days. The way in which hospitals were run then was god-awful. We've come a long way since then." But for all the work and progress made, have we come far enough, and does outside accreditation and regulation do enough as a force for progress? Are these approaches helping to lead the industry or only serving as a brake on progress? Is the health care industry ahead of its standard-setting bodies?

America no longer holds its physicians and health care system in awe. The media produces major investigative pieces continuously. Angry patients and their families have created a blizzard of litigation in the nation's courts. A short surfing expedition on the net turns up countless web addresses on medical litigation, patient rights, and other efforts to blame the industry for its failings. There is a lot of anger out there, and it expresses one central management concern: The standards of America's health system are too low. *Yet nearly all of the hospitals embroiled in litigation were accredited by the JCAHO.*

Biting the Bullet

There is always confusion as to who is responsible, especially when dealing with questions of negligence and malpractice. The argument that many share responsibility for what happens in health care delivery sounds reasonable, among them physicians, nurses, technicians, boards, and suppliers. Nonetheless, although thinking that quality is everybody's responsibility may be comforting, ultimately the responsibility must be borne by health care CEOs and their management teams. What happens inside organizations is what management permits to happen, even if by abdication. To argue otherwise would be sophistry at its worst. It is not the JCAHO's responsibility to produce quality care, it is management's.

Government and hospital leaders first delegated the establishment of accreditation standards to the JCAHO to help with Medicare, but the role of the JCAHO expanded in an effort to meet wider needs. Although there are advantages to having a set of common standards across the industry, JCAHO should not be responsible for the levels of current standards or adherence by individual hospitals to them. Achieving acceptable standards of care is always and only the responsibility of the organization's leaders, for although responsibility can be delegated to the departments, nurses, and doctors, accountability cannot.

What needs to be examined is whether management can rely on outside regulations and inspections as the basis for operational control. If there is value in these historical approaches, corrective actions might simply be a matter of improving existing methods, but if this approach is basically invalid, management should move on to something else. Immense effort and cost have been poured into JCAHO as a regulatory mechanism. But does accreditation work?

Criticisms of the JCAHO

Among the severest critics of the JCAHO has been the watchdog group Public Citizen. This group has a reputation for knowing the facts and speaking out on a wide range of issues in health and public policy. Public Citizen's conclusion about JCAHO accreditation is this (Dame and Wolfe, 1996, p. 37): "We recommend that the Department of Health and Human Services propose, and Congress pass, legislation to repeal 42 U.S.C. § 1395bb, which 'deems' JCAHO-accredited hospitals to meet the conditions of participation in Medicare and Medicaid. HCFA should seek authorization and funding to contract with state agencies to annually survey all participating hospitals to determine compliance with Medicare and Medicaid requirements." Public Citizen reaches the conclusion that JCAHO accreditation is worthless for both public policy and operational reasons.

Failure of Public Policy

What are the points of legitimate questioning as to the effectiveness of JCAHO accreditation? As Public Citizen sees it, these are the main issues:

Conflict of interest. The JCAHO is dominated by the industry it is supposed to regulate. It is governed by a twenty-eight-member board of commissioners primarily representing the industry; twenty-one representatives come from the American College of Physicians, American College of Surgeons, the American Hospital Association, the American Medical Association, and the American Dental Association. (There are also six public representatives and one at-large nursing representative.) The political pressure to meet the needs of these groups is seen by Public Citizen as setting aside the needs of the public. An example of how this potential problem could manifest itself is in board members participating in JCAHO committees that make important decisions, including "the ultimate accreditation status of specific hospitals" (Dame and Wolfe, 1996, p. ix).

Hospitals, not patients, are JCAHO's Customers. Customers of the JCAHO are the hospitals it accredits, not the public at large, which has little or no influence over JCAHO decisions. The organization received $58.7 million in survey fees (Burda, 1994) from its organizational Customers in 1993; according to Public Citizen's logic, money talks. The question of what JCAHO's role should be is called into question when the needs of a hospital organization are put before the needs of the public's safety. The bottom line appears to be that the organization's interests are served, not the public's. The perception grows that enforcement is not happening, and that the JCAHO is only a paper tiger operating in an industry where patients' lives are on the line. As Public Citizen sees it, the JCAHO does not treat hospitals as entities to be regulated, but as Customers to be served and kept satisfied. (A similar criticism was leveled at the Federal Aviation Agency and the National Transport Safety Board in 1996 after a series of air disasters. These agencies were seen as being too cozy with the airline industry by promoting its interests at the same time it was supposed to be regulating airline safety.)

The JCAHO does not meet standards of public accountability. The JCAHO reveals little information regarding the state of its findings; it protects its hospital Customers by limiting and suppressing the information it shares with the media. Further, unlike public agencies, there are no hearings or open meetings to solicit comments, nor is there free access to documents. Enforcement of regulations takes precedence over satisfying hospital Customers.

Points of Operational Failure

In addition to the public policy concerns, critics of the JCAHO cite these problems:

Nearly everyone gets accredited. Possible decisions on accreditation are *accreditation with commendation, accreditation, accreditation with type I recommendations, conditional accreditation,* or *nonaccreditation/denial of accreditation.* On this five-point scale, four positions are passing, and the public is told only whether the hospital is accredited. In 1994 only seven hospitals were denied accreditation by the JCAHO; none were denied in 1995. Basically this means that with few exceptions, any hospital that asks for accreditation gets it. The process is nonexclusionary.

The survey process has problems. Anyone with any management experience would raise an eyebrow at the notion that sufficient monitoring of quality consists of reviewing 700 standards (in the typical JCAHO visit) by a team of three to four visitors over two to five days every three years. To make it worse, surveys are announced far in advance, thus giving hospital staff time to clean up (a commonplace happening). Would any other business go three years between operational audits? Would the military announce in advance when the inspector general would be arriving?

Scoring systems have been weakened. Over time it has become easier for hospitals to achieve a higher level of accreditation. This problem has been occurring for some time, as evidenced by an escalating average *grid score,* an overall score summarizing survey results out of a possible total of 100 points. In 1989 the average hospital grid score was 75.5. The average rose steadily in succeeding years to reach 89.9 in 1995.

To the extent that accreditation is seen as worthless or not credible, hospitals that try to benefit by advertising their accreditation may find it counterproductive. If the current process is indeed flawed, it may help to explain why the problem of quality of care persists. But even if these problems were corrected, would it change the results?

The Role of State Regulation

It may be time to rethink the practice of granting "deemed status" to JCAHO-accredited hospitals as a way to meet state licensure and federal Medicare/Medicaid requirements. Currently, the Health Care Financing Administration (HCFA) and a number of state agencies conduct their own "random" surveys following JCAHO accreditation. "In 1993, 33 percent of the hospitals surveyed failed to meet one or more Medicare conditions of participation, and for the prior six years, from one-fifth to over one-third of the hospitals sampled failed to meet one or more conditions" (Dame and Wolfe, 1996, p. ix).

As a way to improve the validity of what accreditation is supposed to accomplish, HCFA is considering having HCFA and state representatives accompany JCAHO surveyors. Supposedly, this would allow HCFA to see the same situations that the surveyors are evaluating, thus allowing them to evaluate both the institution and the JCAHO process. But the picture of inspectors inspecting inspectors inspecting inspectors inspecting doers just doesn't sound like the best approach. As the old saying goes, "If it takes two people to do one person's job, you don't need one of the people."

However that idea works out, it marks an important step. Government is beginning to think about how to avoid mass infusion of tax monies into a health care system with little direct, governmental oversight and for which the JCAHO system is not performing dependably. Philosophically, Americans don't think government does things better, but practically, Americans don't want problems of quality and cost in health care delivery. Perhaps government inspection would be a better alternative—particularly if the track record shows that more errors would be caught.

JCAHO Customer Dissatisfaction

Although the criticism that the JCAHO is too close to their hospital Customers is a concern in terms of standards management, those same Customers are terribly disenchanted with the JCAHO. In 1994 the Arkansas Hospital Association gave active consideration of mass withdrawal of its members from JCAHO accreditation, and St. Mary's Hospital of Rogers, Arkansas did just that. St. Mary's estimated its savings at $170,000 a year by substituting annual Medicare surveys for the JCAHO procedure (*Modern Healthcare*, May 2, 1994). That hospital Customers have been unhappy about the JCAHO approach to accreditation is an understatement:

> Hospitals grumble about the expense, the time, and effort associated with the accreditation process, and over the past few years several state hospital associations have considered whether their members should withdraw from the JCAHO altogether.[1] In 1994,

[1] State hospital associations in Arkansas, California, Florida, New York, Ohio, Texas, and Wisconsin even formed a coalition to exchange information on alternatives to the JCAHO accreditation process (*Modern Healthcare*, December 19, 1994, p. 2).

the hospitals' growing dissatisfaction culminated in a public display when the AHA announced a "crisis of confidence in the Joint Commission" and stated that substantive change was necessary. In its statement, the AHA criticized the JCAHO for a fundamental lack of responsiveness to the needs of hospitals and their medical staffs, and urged the JCAHO to reassess its future role, "with particular sensitivity to issues of role conflict and Customer focus." [Statement on the Joint Commission, American Hospital Association Board of Trustees, December 19, 1994 (Dame and Wolfe, 1996, p. 17)]

Changes at JCAHO

Belatedly the accrediting agency has been moving to improve its system. Its internally designed IMS standards proved impossible for the industry to accept. The Oryx replacement, in which performance outcomes, not processes, are measured, is philosophically a change in the right direction. Consumer advocates will hardly be pleased, however, since only a few measures are required that cover the patient population. Although that's a legitimate concern, it is probably realistic operationally. And though the percentage is small currently, the number of measures and percentage of patients covered is to increase over several years. It remains to be seen whether a number of issues can be worked out, including the validity of measures supplied differently by a wide range of measurement vendors, and the question of cost, which can be particularly difficult for small and rural hospitals. The Maryland Hospital Association's Quality Indicator Project won the most clients out of the 344 systems competing in 1998, thus suggesting that it is becoming a de facto standard among measurement service providers (J. Moore, 1998c).

In another development, the Joint Commission on Accreditation of Health Care Organizations, the National Committee for Quality Assurance, and the American Medical Accreditation Program are attempting to deal with the question of proliferating and nonaligned standards. By jointly sponsoring the Performance Measurement Coordinating Council, they hope to reach consensus on standards, avoid redundancies, and make sure that different areas of practice are covered. What path this effort will ultimately take is unclear, but addressing the explosion of standards and their measures is needed.

Another positive development is the use by JCAHO of *sentinel events*—situations that led to death, serious injury, or the risk thereof—to determine the weaknesses in existing procedures, systems, and habits. The controversy surrounding this aggressive management approach concerns whether such sentinel events will put the organization's accreditation status at risk. Sentinel events need to be reported directly by hospitals so that all may learn and change, rather than waiting for them to appear as scandals in the press. For the four years from 1995 through 1998, only 374 sentinel events were reviewed by the JCAHO. Yet even this small sample of the much larger universe of thousands of misadventures revealed that only three of the twenty-two problem categories accounted for 168 (45 percent) of the events: patient suicide (80 cases), medication error (59 cases), and operative or postoperative complication (29 cases) (Helfrick, 1999). Sentinel event reporting can be an extremely powerful tool as the industry moves forward.

A Reflection on Critics

In any review of the JCAHO, one has to critique the critics as well. Is a mind game being played by some health care organizations? Do they criticize the JCAHO while permitting themselves to run a sloppy ship? The difficulties of running hospitals and health systems can be tremendously stressful and frustrating. It is easy to lash out at the JCAHO, perhaps even use them and other outside factors as scapegoats. The truth is that the agency tries hard, does a lot of good (according to its fans), and is caught up in the turbulence of the times. Even granting that JCAHO has been behind the change wave, the industry might benefit from less blaming and more rethinking as to how things need to be done from now on.

The Future of the JCAHO

So where do we go from here? One suggestion came in reaction to yet another squabble between the AHA and several state hospital associations with the JCAHO over its Oryx performance measurement program. *Modern Healthcare* was scathing in its criticism, but on target in its message: "In its forty-eight years, the Joint Commission has never based accreditation on how well a hospital takes care of its patients. Five decades is too long for such a lapse. The industry and the Joint Commission should drop the infighting and finish the overdue work. If they can't do it, somebody else, like the government, for instance, just might" (McLaughlin, 1999).

Are we continuing to support something that appears good on its surface but in truth is a sham, well intentioned though it may be? There is increasing consumer demand for quality information regarding health providers. *Consumer's Guide to Hospitals* shows hospital-by-hospital death rates by major surgical procedure (Center for the Study of Services, 1994). It has been highlighted in recent American Association of Retired Persons (AARP) publications, and represents the voice of consumerism. The public wants to know relative quality and cost data by hospital and procedure. Consumers see as arrogant the efforts by health professionals who fight disclosure and debate the data's accuracy or the public's ability to understand it. The public seems less interested in JCAHO accreditation than in seeing performance outcomes.

Respected thinker Clark Havighurst (1992) called for competition for the JCAHO as one way to better reach quality goals. Now, when new thinking is sorely needed, competitive approaches should not just be allowed, they should be required. The conclusion may be painful but it must be drawn: The JCAHO's original purposes and methodologies have been surpassed by the current need for a more direct approach to judging excellence among health providers. In its current configuration the JCAHO is at best anachronistic. The industry cannot afford a fogged illusion that accreditation procedures are protecting quality.

Confusing Means with Ends

Part of what is wrong with the three historical approaches to assuring standards in health care (certification, licensure, and accreditation) is that they share a flawed set of assumptions about how management really works. Repeatedly proven in the management literature is the fact that one must focus on end results, not on approach or third party endorsement. Focusing on results means first setting a goal or objective, then defining the measures that tell whether you made it. Only then does one turn to the question of how we're going to get there, and what actions and strategies will be pursued. The dictum remains: One manages by objectives, or one doesn't manage.

This common failure to understand that success is in the results, not in the process, was pointedly described by Robert Schaffer and Harvey Thomson (1992), widely regarded for their work in organizational change management. In the *Harvard Business Review*, they describe the faulty thinking process that has too long been followed by leaders and standard setters in health care.

> The performance improvement efforts of many companies have as much impact on operational and financial results as a ceremonial rain dance has on the weather. While some companies constantly improve measurable performance, in many others managers continue to dance round and round the campfire—exuding faith and dissipating energy.
>
> This "rain dance" is the ardent pursuit of activities that sound good, look good, and allow managers to feel good—but in fact contribute little or nothing to bottom line performance. . . . At the heart of these programs, which we call "activity-centered," is a fundamentally flawed logic that confuses ends with means, processes with outcomes. . . . The momentum for activity-centered programs continues to accelerate even though there is virtually no evidence to justify the flood of investment. Just the opposite: there is plenty of evidence that the rewards from these activities are illusory. [Robert H. Schaffer and Harvey A. Thomson, "Successful Change Programs Begin with Results," *Harvard Business Review* (Jan.-Feb., 1992), pp. 80–89. Used by permission of the publisher.]

The activity-centered fallacy has the cards stacked against it because these efforts are not keyed to specific results, they're too large or too diffused, results are treated as a four-letter word, and they have delusional measurements. On the latter, Schaffer and Thomson observe: "The Malcolm Baldrige National Quality Award encourages such [activity versus results] practices by devoting only 180 points out of a possible 1,000 points to quality results. The award gives high marks to companies that demonstrate outstanding quality processes without always demanding that the current products and services be equally outstanding" (Schaffer and Thomson, 1992, p. 82).

The movement to extend the Baldrige award to health care might be managerially useful in that it can energize an organization around quality goals. However, the Baldrige award has had mixed reviews about its criteria and the unanswered question of whether its defined criteria have anything to do with running a successful business. The classic case in point was Florida Power and Light, whose CEO, John Hudiburg, was fired after winning both Japan's Deming prize and the Baldrige. The embarrassment was total, with front page stories appearing in both *Fortune* ("Is the Baldrige Overblown?" 1991) and *Forbes* ("A Hero Without a Company," 1991). The reason: Customer complaints were higher than all other utilities in the state, as was the cost of the electricity provided. Florida Power and Light won prizes, but ruined its business.

Both the JCAHO and health care leaders need to move toward a focus on results that is primarily fixed on outcome measures. That is clearly the direction that employers and payers are moving in as well. We can no longer listen to those who endlessly chant "process, process, process" and tell us to wait patiently for years to see the results. As one CEO said, "In twenty years of working with hospital boards, I never met one that would buy a results horizon of ten years. They want results now." This wise view of the world matches what the professional practice of management is all about —producing real results and producing them quickly. What we need to shake off is the mindset of the religiously orthodox who think they know the answers, and that all we have to do is have faith and be more dedicated to the "right" steps. What we really need is more dedication to empirical results.

Looking Beyond JCAHO for Standards

In 1993 JCAHO declared that it would welcome any other organization that would care to offer accreditation services. That call has apparently been answered, but not in the way they anticipated. There has been an unprecedented explosion in information gathering regarding clinical quality, costs, even the track records of individual practitioners. As this body of knowledge grows, no single agency will be able to encompass and judge it all or maintain a monopoly in judging the organizations that produce it.

Accreditation is at best an outsider's secondary opinion regarding quality, whereas patient care outcomes, Customer satisfaction ratings, and cost of services are primary indicators of correct performance. That is certainly the conclusion being drawn by consumers, the nation's employers, and the payers who are the servants of the former two groups. Accreditation will continue as a service into the near future, but its value will lessen as outcomes and results achieved through correctly designed best practices, not accreditation, become the rightful yardsticks by which organizational effectiveness and patient treatment are judged. Perhaps JCAHO will evolve into the premier provider of best practices information.

At heart, consumers don't care about accreditation: They simply want assurance that their health care provider is producing affordable quality care. What sources, other than accreditation, are available to judge that, and how might they be organized to better serve market needs? Who really writes the standards that must be met to prove we deserve to stand in the winner's circle?

The Standards Within

Why do people who don't deliver health care think they know enough about work they've never done, in places they've never seen, to tell those who are on the field what they should do? Although regulators, academics, and payers represent important viewpoints, those views have to be placed in the practical limits of the real world of managing. What is it truly possible to do here? And are we listening to the voices within our organization? Is it possible that too much attention has been paid to advice from the outside, and too little attention given to the people within our health care organizations—both the people who do the work and the Customers whom they serve? Rather than listening to "Monday morning quarterbacks," let's go to the people on the field to understand the direction that standards need to take.

The Supreme Court of Customer Opinion

Who sets standards? There are many sources, but let's begin with the patient. Patients have their own set of standards and expectations. An organization is in peril when it ignores its Customer and doesn't measure its performance against Customer expectations. When what Customers expect (courtesy, timeliness, accuracy) does not happen, there is a gap between their level of expectation and the existing level of reality. This gap creates a negative evaluation of their experience. When the hospital is not as clean as the Customer's home, you're going to hear about it, as you deserve, for in this regard the patient has higher standards than your organization. When the food is cold or bad and the Customer tells you, there's another reminder that things need to be done better. Said one executive, "I don't view patient comments as complaints to be resisted but as free consulting on how to improve my business."

When Customers experience a level of reality that is equal to their level of expectation, there is satisfaction, but it's not going to be seen as extraordinary. Only when the level of reality is greater than the level of expectation will there be an eye-opening, positively charged response. Meeting Customer expectations (standards) is the minimum necessary to stay in business. Exceeding expectations is what represents competitive advantage—what Bill Gonzalez, CEO of Spectrum Health System, a "Top 100 Hospitals" winner, calls "wow service, miracle service." We're going to have to go beyond the past definitions of good service to a new level of unfailing service—not to an extremism of luxuries provided, but to an extremism of attention to work detail and constant respect in relationships.

What is wonderful about the individual observations and the collective opinions of Customers is that they represent thousands of perceptions about how you're doing—from intelligent and successful people, from hurting and grieving people, but always from people who want you to get an "A" that day. They see things in the organization you don't; they see the staff in ways you don't. They are in a position to help you, if you will listen. And listen you will if you truly understand that Customer standards are currently the single most reliable guide available to success.

Some would like to draw the line at that statement. They argue that Customers probably are good judges of administrative procedures and other nonclinical aspects of their care, but that they are unable to detect faults in their medical care. Although patients usually are not expert in treatment procedures, they are expert in the body they've carried around for a lifetime. They may not know the anatomical labels, but they can tell where it hurts, when, and following what kind of physical movement. Studies have repeatedly shown that patients are often highly accurate in knowing they have a problem, and that physicians who are expert diagnosticians typically spend more time asking the patient questions about their condition than their less effective counterparts. This was borne out in a study done by the Physician Insurers Association, which found that breast cancer accounted for more medical malpractice claims and lawsuits than any other condition, and that delayed diagnosis was the leading cause. In 70 percent of the cases, women had discovered a suspicious lump and gone to their doctor, but the physician had dismissed their complaint or delayed taking action (Morrissey, 1995). The primary recommendation from the study was to take more time and give more weight to patient complaints. It would seem that even clinical standards and technical protocols would benefit from some form of Customer input or evaluation, even though caregivers remain the primary decision makers.

To what patient reports and requests need we listen? Most hospitals break out their surveys by inpatient, outpatient, outpatient surgery, and emergency room areas. But beyond these groupings are others that may yield rich treasures. Research has already determined that men have expectations different from women, older people different from younger. Indeed, there are particular needs, expectations, and standards that each patient type has of their health care experience. Nearly everyone expects to be treated with courtesy and respect, but the winning organization will go beyond these basic universals. With deeper information, changes in work systems become intelligently driven.

There's also the question of frequency. A quarterly summary isn't nearly as helpful as a shorter survey of what occurred last week. Management control of operations is increased when data are real-time or at least recent. Holy Cross Hospital in Chicago tries to identify, by department each week, issues needing attention based on the previous week's results.

But survey data can be "old and cold" and often go unused in America's hospitals. Data often reside in voluminous reports that never reach those doing the work, or remain in a format that is impossible to use. It is possible to get a good handle on this problem, today, by direct action. Caregivers can visit patients and ask family members how the organization is doing. Hospitals of the new era often use an adopt-a-patient program. Each patient receives daily visits from a staff member during each day of their stay, not as a direct caregiver, but as a friend. The impact on staff and patients is wonderful, and the learning gained by the organization tremendous. Although I believe in the rigorous collection of data, I believe even more in responding right now to direct instruction from Customers.

Can patients truly judge quality? Is there any validity to their experience? Absolutely. Is there any better measure or source of standards? No, nothing else is even close. What's the goal of any business? Isn't it to satisfy its Customers at the highest possible level? Meet their standards, their expectation that nothing less than the best will be provided. The Customer becomes the central measure of the organization's performance.

How far removed were some health care providers from this simple business principle of paying attention to the Customer? The press reports were everywhere as Customers fought to get laws requiring a Patient Bill of Rights. That this was a hotly contested issue years ago clearly indicated how far out of touch some health care providers were. Effective managements will actively engage in listening to the Customer. (For much more on this topic, read *Total Customer Satisfaction* by S. Sherman, 1998).

I suggest this goal: 95 percent of Customers will say, "This is the best hospital I've ever received care from." The Customer becomes a true measure of the organization's performance.

Physicians as Standards Source

Who else sets standards worth meeting? Ask physicians what they think of working in hospitals that can't supply lab information quickly enough, that mislabel blood bags, don't supply qualified staff, or alienate their patients. Something's wrong when medical practitioners' standards are higher than those good enough for an organization to pass accreditation. When physician practice is compromised because of a poorly responsive organization, it's time to upgrade what we're doing.

A mistake that health care organizations make too often is treating physicians with kid gloves instead of grabbing their hand in the grip of partnership. When asked whether yet another survey of physician needs should be run, one takeover hospital executive with a track record to be proud of exploded, "Absolutely not! You've surveyed them endlessly for years. Start turning information into results; take action on what they've been repeatedly telling us." Said a physician leader bluntly, "If you want to make the doctors happy, stop pissing off their patients. It gets tiresome to take it in the ear on everything the hospital's doing wrong every time you walk in to see your patient."

A debate has been raging as to the proper balance between managed care and a physician's right to practice medicine as she chooses. Clearly, costs must and can be cut by moving toward standardized best practices—clinical care protocols. And some physicians produce poor quality and costs, and action should be taken to alter their poor professional practice. But HMOs and managed care organizations have often made ignorant and ill-informed decisions that they zealously administer. About half the states have now enacted laws that prevent managed care organizations, and medical groups who benefit from managed care contracts, from retaliating against physicians who give their patients appropriate care. In commenting on a jury finding that physicians were being muzzled and harassed by managed care, Miles Zaremski, a Chicago lawyer and former head of an American Bar Association medicine and law committee, said, "The message is exceedingly clear: patient care over profits and medicine over money. This message is being sent by representatives of the American public, the jury" (Brandon, 1998). As the market speaks, payers and physicians are being told to work out a new balance for a win-win solution.

As physicians reemerge from the distraction of the managed care debate and resume their proper leadership over patient care, health care organizations will increasingly turn to them as partners in determining how best care should be delivered. Physicians can be thought of as patient agents who are particularly knowledgeable about all the clinical workings and process problems in the house. Physician Customers have the behind-the-scene understandings that patients lack. The physician becomes a palpable measure of the organization. Their involvement is critical in defining clinical protocols, standardizing formulary, and redefining the proper balance of professional practice in the midst of limited resources.

In the necessary drive to please payers, executives must broker new relationships with physicians. Physician treatment practices do need to change. But primacy must be placed on the relationship with physicians as partners while reducing costs without damaging quality. These two necessary outcomes are not mutually exclusive; only a short-sighted view of cost reduction would make it so. While these issues are worked out, trust the collective judgment of internal patients' agents to provide numerous suggestions for needed change. Their standards of what is required is a necessary part of the equation for winning.

I suggest this goal: 95 percent of physicians will say, "This is the best organization I've ever practiced medicine in." The physician becomes a measure of the organization.

Staff Associates Are Essential

Are there other sources of standards better than those of accrediting agencies? Each day hundreds of thousands of health care workers trudge off to work, work they have done for years and invested years of study to learn how to do. Every single one of them knows something that needs to be improved. Their individual and collective voices should be shaping our organizations because they *are* the organization. As one veteran manager put it: "If anyone thinks that Associates aren't the most important part of the organization, test it by sending them all home and see how much patient care gets delivered." Who cares more about quality and Customers than the people who are giving their lives to this work? What does it say when we listen more to consultant outsiders advising us about standards than we listen to those whose personal standards and values—and professional standards and values— are better than anything that's going on around them? Associates should set standards for the organization. In each department, let each member of the team be asked what the standards should be. Invariably staff push for higher levels of performance. The reason is simple: No one wants to give their lives to mediocrity.

To use these individual experiences and organization sensors effectively, management must find ways to allow Associates' ideation to flow and then gather this collective wisdom. One key measure is surveys on staff attitudes and opinions. In recent years these surveys have become more precise in spotting workplace issues, safety concerns, areas needing improvement, and team needs.

I suggest this goal: 95 percent of Associates will say, "This is the best organization I've ever worked in." The Associate becomes a measure of the organization.

Competition

We often refer to competition as meaning another organization in our market. But competition isn't just about the other guy. To compete is to be in a contest, usually for a prize, and usually with a team. A strong competitor can help us, because we know we have to stay on top of our game or be bested by them. Indeed, it is difficult for a health care organization to get better without a competitor. But there are other meanings to competition.

All health care organizations are competing against illness and death. We measure these events' severity and frequency and set goals. One of the problems for world-record holders in track is that they have no one else to compete against. They have to compete against themselves, striving for a "personal best." Setting up internal competitions against our own statistics is another way to raise the bar—and to achieve our personal best.

Internal competition between departments or organizations within a system is another way management can spark the desire to win. This tactic takes some consideration because we don't want internal competition to interfere with interunit cooperation. Find an element with some comparability between units—number of training hours, number of ideas per person, or Customer satisfaction ratings. People love to win, so keep the atmosphere friendly, not pressured, and have some fun with it.

The Standards Outside

Outside regulators, agencies, and organizations are issuing standards that can be an important part of the success equation for providers. If designed properly, these can become governance mechanisms that lead rather than hinder higher performance.

Government Representing People

Pennsylvania was the first state to release report cards on hospital performance, and it has done so annually since 1989. Florida has now joined in and evaluates 202 hospitals on expected mortality rates, prices, and lengths of stay. The report cards evaluate fifteen clinical service areas, including cardiac and general surgery, obstetrics, pediatrics, and urology. Hospitals are graded as being either in the top 15 percent of all hospitals, the bottom 15 percent, or the middle 70 percent. As one might suppose, hospital managements are either pleased or displeased based on their rating. The data are expected to be used by consumers and payers (Greene, 1996).

Massachusetts took the lead in publishing detailed information on the states' 30,000 licensed physicians, including felony convictions, charges in which a physician pleaded no contest, any disciplinary actions, revocation or restriction of hospital privileges, and medical malpractice findings. Although other states publish some limited information, Massachusetts has put together a comprehensive picture available from a single source. Though *Modern Healthcare* reports that not all physicians are happy about this approach, the pressure of severe consumer agitation on the issue made it "hard to fight the inevitable" ("Massachusetts to Publish Doc Profile Data," 1996).

By 1998, nearly all hospitals had joined in the effort, using the same questionnaire and jointly released results. Sponsored by the Massachusetts Health Quality Partnership, a consortium representing hospitals, employers, doctors, and insurers, the survey was conducted by the Picker Institute. The process has matured to the point that the hospitals all agreed to release the findings, not to use the findings in advertising, and not to publicly criticize the methodology. The media has also matured, and coverage is described as educational and responsible, with no slamming of lower-rated organizations (J. Moore, 1998a). In this open environment all parties are able to focus on making improvement that is to the benefit of all.

Under this approach, the state does not seek to change hospital or physician behavior but simply to provide information so that the free market forces put the squeeze on poor operators and reward those with better track records. Other states will probably follow. The veil of secrecy is clearly coming down, and the argument that the "ignorant consumer" can't judge these matters is a sophistry and arrogance that is part of health care's past. The course to pursue is to create organizations that look good in these rating systems, a minimal standard.

Medicare and Medicaid regulations continue to expand as dispensers of government money seek to get more results for the tax money expended. In a number of states, health care executives have abandoned JCAHO accreditation in favor of state surveys, which they find more thorough and affordable.

HCFA is posting survey reports of the quality of nursing homes on Medicare's Internet site. Consumers can get information about a particular nursing home just by entering its name. Any violations cited by the certification agencies are posted, along with a comparison to the average number of violations per nursing home in the state (Gardner, 1998). Although this is not a particularly happy event for some organizations, it represents government's serving taxpayers and may be a model of dealing with hospitals and health care professionals in the future.

Government needs to rethink its role in regulation. In dealing with the turbulence of an exploding knowledge industry like health care, structured regulations need to be replaced with direction and incentives for those meeting higher standards and moving toward standardized best practices in all departments. Government leaders can assist this process of evolution by sponsoring initiatives and alliances that bring together major players around proposals for national clearinghouses, professional endorsements of standards and approved practices, and schemes for awarding attainment of these new levels. Government regulations aimed only at protecting the public against health care failure are shortsighted and poorly aimed. Standards now must foster the attainment of higher levels of performance.

NCQA and HEDIS

The National Committee for Quality Assurance (NCQA), as part of its accreditation and evaluation of managed-care plans, has moved to the forefront in measuring outcomes of health care performance. The Health Plan Employer Data and Information Set (HEDIS) is a set of seventy-five measures (as of 1997) that cover clinical performance outcomes and financial, service, and access measures important to purchasers in making contracting decisions. Another thirty measures are in the testing stage, and the outlook is for expansion of this effort to gather and disseminate data. About 330 health plans, approximately half of the nation's total, are currently using HEDIS to report their performance to large employers and other purchasers (Morrissey, 1996a). NCQA will reportedly be incorporating HEDIS information in their evaluation process beginning in 1999.

Data tell the story. It's been said that the first law of the universe is the almighty dollar bill. Employers and payers continue to require more outcome data because the health bill is still escalating. The more we can identify patterns of care and cost, the more intelligently we can manage. One effect information reporting is having is to streamline and standardize health care's information systems. What is more important, patient outcomes are benefiting. At HealthPartners, child immunizations rose to 89 percent in 1996 from 54 percent four years earlier (Morrissey, 1996a). Finally, under HMO prodding, many more providers are following standardized procedures or clinical guidelines with proven outcomes (Kertesz, 1996). According to a study released in February 1996, six out of ten employers already pick plans by using HEDIS and accreditation by NCQA (Jaklevic, 1996).

Resistance to HEDIS has been based on the difficult nature of meeting the reporting requirements, the accuracy and relevance of the data, and the dreaded effect it can have on payments. Resentment has been expressed toward HMOs and other agents of managed care. At a recent meeting, one HMO spokesman said to a roomful of hospital executives, "Don't be mad at us. We're simply doing, and we're going to continue to do, what big business wants." The loud wailing from certain quarters led *Modern Healthcare* to pronounce in an editorial:

> With the new [HEDIS] measures . . . health plans are about to become accountable for proof of good performance in both acute and chronic care. Such guidelines are helping transform health care from a cottage industry to a mature, fully coordinated, trillion-dollar enterprise.
>
> Unfortunately, the transition often resembles a holy war. Individuals and groups struggling to assure their own economic survival. . . .
>
> Providers that wish to thrive in a managed-care environment must be able to prove how well patients treated in their facilities fared. They must do it with data, not vague generalities. It will require providers working closely with health plans, rather than trashing one another. When the day comes—and it soon will—that all plans and providers are measured by standardized yardsticks, then quality organizations can stand out with assurances they provide their communities high-quality, affordable care. [Editorial, "New HEDIS Measures Give Providers Chance to Mature," *Modern Healthcare,* July 22, 1996, p. 26. Used by permission of the publisher]

NCQA has also been affecting performance outcomes by requiring an HMO seeking accreditation to have a proper physician credentialing process. This one aspect alone constitutes 25 percent of the accreditation decision, thus quickly driving out the "aberrant, unlicensed or poorly certified providers, or those with poor performance." Evidence is also mounting that the median court settlement in malpractice cases has dropped from nearly $500,000 in 1991 to $325,000 in 1995 largely because of increased pressure to remove these poor performers (Kertesz, 1996).

In what is an exciting development, a number of hospital executives have experimentally begun using NCQA measurements (designed for HMOs) as areas to measure in their own performance.

g is that if payers are going to be judged on certain
e same criteria or measured areas are going to pass
ne way or another to providers. By looking at a similar
rns, they get the jump on competitors who aren't think-
the narrow confines of the accreditation box. These
early adopters might be a harbinger of things to come. Perhaps
NCQA will evolve into a direct accrediting agency for providers,
thus allowing a more consistent set of standards from payer to
provider to patient.

HMOs and Patient Satisfaction Measures

Employers and their agent HMOs are now putting real pressure
on providers to measure patient satisfaction. In the early days,
HMOs were reputed to be only interested in cost—their initial
starting point. As development of the data has continued, quality
outcomes measures have been added because employers want to
be able to steer their employees to providers who won't alienate
employees into a negative backlash. Finally, an increased use of
patient satisfaction indices has emerged, partly because variations
in price and geographic coverage have ceased being a competitive
factor in some markets. Satisfaction thus becomes a competitive
distinction. And there is mounting evidence that patients who are
unhappy with a provider hospital or physician are more than willing to change health plans. Indeed, health plans have a real Customer retention problem. The answer is to get the full picture of
cost, quality, and service satisfaction, which allows payers to steer
users to best overall providers. The net effect on providers: Either
move upwards in attaining performance standards or be economically starved to death.

Blue Cross of California now requires hospitals to provide Customer satisfaction data. Reportedly, employers in states like California, Ohio, and Wisconsin are sharing this information with
employees to assist them in picking providers. The American Medical Association reports it will incorporate patient satisfaction measures in its new accreditation program for physicians. The Pacific
Business Group on Health and the Medical Quality Commission
would like to see their survey, the Physician Value Check, become

the state standard in California (Jaklevic, 1995). Although most measures are still nonstandardized and too widely variant to allow comparison, the patient's perception will become increasingly important in judging providers.

Key industries are learning how to direct their substantial clout in the standards arena. Results were released for the first time in 1999 of a joint effort by the Big Three automakers and the United Auto Workers to study health care quality. This report card was based on the National Committee for Quality Assurance HEDIS data on HMO performance. The Rand Corporation also evaluated the results to ensure comparability across plan providers who were evaluated on the following:

- Customer satisfaction and access
- Preventive care
- Illness recovery
- Treatment of chronic conditions

The rating scale was three points: *significantly above average, average,* and *significantly below average.* Approximately 20 percent of the plan received *significantly above average* ratings. The report cards will be made available to the automakers' employees and will have substantial economic impact, at least in regions where there are competing plans.

Along the path toward more open sharing of information will be many setbacks. The Cleveland Clinic Health System, with nine of its ten hospitals participating, dropped out of the Cleveland Health Quality Choice Program, which had been sponsored by a coalition of provider and employer organizations. The organization reported that the data it was reporting along with other providers on mortality and length of stay were not useful or understandable to most consumers. At the same time, Moody's turned negative in its ratings on the $630 million of debt held by the clinic and the operating loss being experienced by the system (Jaklevic, 1999). Staying the course with quality reporting might have been a better strategy. Industry rotation, whereby an industry's leaders are replaced by a new generation of more aggressive organizations, often occurs precisely at the point when the old leader loses its edge in the standards game.

Bogus Measures of Performance

The health care industry is still maturing in terms of how it measures organizational performance. All of us to want to win, cross
the finish line ahead of the others, and find that our work has mattered. But no one would want this under false pretenses or be
happy with a counterfeit prize. As Michael Jordan said in 1998,
heading into the National Basketball Association playoffs after yet
another winning season: "It don't mean a thing if you don't have
the ring." Although winning the prize is a great goal, there are
counterfeit prizes abounding in health care. Their presence distracts from the real playoff effort of meeting higher performance
levels. Examples of bogus prizes include the following:

• "America's Best Hospitals." Each year *U.S. News and World
Report* publishes a list of "America's Best Hospitals." According to
one report, that list of 126 hospital finalists was culled from a list
of 1,961 hospitals. Hardly representative, according to *U.S. News
and World Report,* "to be considered, a hospital had to be a member of the Council of Teaching Hospitals, be affiliated with a medical school, or have nine or more of eighteen specific items of
technology." Further, one-third of the total score rested on the
frail basis of reputation ("America's Best Hospitals: Behind the
Rankings," 1996). A far more damning indictment was published
in the *Journal of the American Medical Association,* which concluded
that the *U.S. News* ranking isn't much more than a popularity contest with little to do with concrete measures of patient care (*Journal of the American Medical Association,* 1997 [cited in *Modern
Healthcare,* 1997]).

• Vendor prizes. Entirely too many awards from vendors are
held up as evidence of real achievement. At best such prizes are
based on some anecdotal or surface indication, but more likely
they are more a statement of economic connection and profits-
derived than a measure of true merit. A far more valuable offering
might come from a vendors' conference: Learning what's working
elsewhere is far more valuable than receiving a phony prize.

• Association awards. Often given because of active participation or political connection, the plaques line the walls of our
health care organizations. But the real questions are, Did patients
get better, did costs go down, did quality improve? These are un-

comfortable questions to ask, but they must be asked if we're to get past the frosting and down to substance.

• Accreditation. Various accreditation, certification, and licensure procedures operate within the industry; JCAHO is chief among them. The logic is that the presence of certain qualifying criteria (educational level, hours of continuing education, proper supervision) or processes (organizational structures, policy and procedure manuals, frameworks for decision making) will be correlated to proper and cost-effective care. This argument is faulty, as argued elsewhere in this book. This is not to say there is no value in these approaches for the present, only that they are proving insufficient and must be retooled if they are to be effective in the future.

With those criticisms made, let's be practical. If somebody wants to give your hospital a plaque, take it. Any executive who is offered an award from Baxter or Marriott or *U.S. News* who doesn't take it is an idiot. If you get accreditation with commendation, call in the press. Display it, praise the troops for winning it, make a big deal out of it, have a party. In the struggle to move onward and upward, we can use these opportunities to motivate and teach. But in their hearts, effective leaders know we must find a better way to determine whether we've done the job and done it right.

Where Are Standards Heading?

A standards revolution is occurring. A major rethinking is under way. First, consideration is being given to which existing standards should be recalibrated and used. Second, a number of trends indicate where elevating standards are heading.

Recalibrating Standards

Figure 4.1 suggests that existing sources of standards can be split into old and new camps. The older sources can still be used, but they tend to be minimal standards and not as useful for organizations trying to excel and thrive. Perhaps in time these will be rethought and refurbished into something more meaningful. The newer sources, on which winning managements are focusing, are internal (where wide participation allows for improvements to

Figure 4.1. Sources of Standards.

Old Secondary	New Primary
• JCAHO	• Management (measure)
• State regulators	• Customers (measure)
• Federal regulators	• Physicians (measure)
• Professional societies	• Associates (measure)
• Hospital associations	• Vendors/suppliers
• Industry awards	• • • •
	• Best practices libraries
	• Benchmark organizations
	• NCQA/HEDIS (payers)
	• • • •
	• Top 100 measures?
	• Baldrige award?

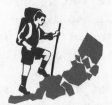

flow), come from outside definers of state-of-the-art best practices, or represent a pursuit toward genuine and tough-to-get prizes.

Trends in Standards Evolution

What may we reasonably expect to see occur with standards in the near future? Here is a list of predictions:

Increased demand for outcomes data. The demand from employers, payers, and consumers for complete information on cost, quality outcomes, and Customer satisfaction scores will continue unabated. We will see the end of secreting clinical care outcomes, protecting the poorly performing practitioner, and hiding outcomes data. In a survey of 368 companies (see Table 4.1) conducted by the Washington Business Group on Health, which represents large employers, it was found that "significantly, employers of all sizes expect to adopt more quality measures in the next two years" (Jaklevic, 1996).

The lower percentages among smaller employers is probably a result of the smaller size of staff to pursue these projects. The large employers will most likely call the tune and establish universal and standardized reporting from all providers.

Table 4.1. Top Ten Future Data Sources.

Data Sources	% Large Employers	% Small Employers
Disease/condition-specific outcomes	32	6
NCQA accreditation status	27	10
Audited report cards	26	6
HEDIS	22	4
Employer-specified performance standards	18	9
Other accreditation status	14	1
Quality improvement initiatives	13	4
Results of consumer satisfaction surveys	12	10
Plan-sponsored practice protocols	12	3
Medical loss ratios	9	2

Sources: Washington Business Group on Health and Watson Wyatt Worldwide, as quoted in Jaklevic (1996).

Outcomes data will be widely shared with the public. Data gained from HEDIS are beginning to be shared with the public, a trend that will gather more momentum as data collection increases and becomes more refined. The Pacific Business Group on Health released information on eleven Los Angeles HMOs, and the North Central Texas HEDIS coalition released information on seven Dallas area health plans. Similar projects occurred in Denver and Pittsburgh (Morrissey, 1996b, p. 33). In the future, in each market, HMO and provider information on quality, access to care, and use of services will appear in the press and on television. The public wants to know this information far more than whether the hospital is accredited.

Business intends to enlist the public as a force for change and to influence specific purchasing decisions in the marketplace. When corporate executives, some of the most achievement-driven people in American culture, saw career ambitions and corporate fortunes placed in jeopardy by rising health costs, it was easy to predict that there would be a counterattack. As G.E.'s Jack Welch said, "Control your destiny or someone else will." Corporate America may not be the only player on the stage, but it is playing a lead role. One recent survey found that 80 percent of employers who offered medical benefits had adopted some form of HMO cost oversight—the question of whether HMOs would succeed is over. The appropriate response now for providers is simply to get the jobs of cost reduction, quality improvement, and Customer satisfaction done.

NCQA may become the national health care accrediting body. NCQA has emerged as the de facto leader in accreditation in the managed care arena. It is highly likely that NCQA accreditation will become the minimum standard that employers use to pick plans. With the health system moving toward a majority of covered lives under managed care, it will make no sense for a plan provider to be accredited by NCQA and a hospital provider to be accredited by JCAHO. Either NCQA standards will be used to accredit hospital providers, in which case JCAHO will cease to exist, or JCAHO will become only an implementing agent for NCQA standards. The latter alternative has already begun, as JCAHO has started to use some NCQA standards. In "computerese," JCAHO may simply become "NCQA compatible."

Increased measurement will force industry improvement. The standard setter in each locale will simply be the organization with the best numbers. Attaining higher performance levels is a stealth weapon in a competitive war. Just as the quality and cost of Japanese cars in the 1970s and 1980s took huge market share and forced a retooling of the American automobile industry, so, too, will health organizations have to compete on quality and cost or face extinction. Once the data are available, lesser providers can run, but they can't hide.

Competition will be redefined. Currently cost is the major battleground of competition, one that many hospitals are still making excuses about. But corporate America learned in the 1980s that good quality and low cost go together. Corporate managers believe that hospitals' high costs are reflective of poor quality and its associated problems. Having been through massive reengineering and restructuring themselves, they know they can provide higher quality at lower cost. Seventy-three percent of employers surveyed don't buy the idea that quality of care suffers because providers are being pressured to keep costs down (Schlesinger and Heskett,

1991). So quality is rapidly becoming the second competitive battleground. Initially *quality* is likely to be defined as "an absence of defects," but the definition will quickly move beyond that to "higher levels of performance."

Experience in other industries suggests that once cost and quality are achieved on a par with competitors, more attention is likely to be paid to Customer satisfaction. It becomes the last untouched area for differentiation. Initially, *satisfaction* is defined as an "absence of irritations" but rapidly moves to "pleased with the total experience." J. D. Powers reported in 1996 that the two cars with highest Customer satisfaction were Lexus and Saturn. Although their products sell at opposite ends of the cost spectrum, both organizations have learned that knowing both stated and unstated Customer expectations, and then exceeding them, is the key to Customer retention. And it is Customer retention more than Customer satisfaction that is the key to long-term success (Morrissey, 1996b).

Measures will be refined. The Foundation for Accountability, an alliance of consumers and health care purchasers, is pushing for "common-sense measures of health care performance. . . . Instead of focusing on complex clinical processes, which typify measures within the health field . . . its measures will attempt to make comparisons possible about results of treatment and overall quality of life" (Schlesinger and Heskett, 1991). Their concept is to get these plain English measures written into payers' contracts with providers and included in HEDIS. The organization's board includes Paul Ellwood, president of the Jackson Hole Group, representatives from HCFA, private sector purchasers of health care, and consumer organizations.

Eventually, specific and detailed knowledge of provider performance will be translated into ratings that are simple to understand. Why would the public want to know more detailed information about the Four Seasons Hotel in Chicago once it knows that it is rated five stars and voted the best big-city hotel by frequent business travelers? Similar shorthand ratings may be an eventual outcome of the period ahead. Once we have figured out which criteria are essential, it will be possible to reach summary conclusions more quickly and easily than we can now.

Should the Top 100 Hospitals Be Your Goal?

As an illustration of the power of higher standards, consider the impact it would have if your hospital was a winner of Top 100 Hospitals status. Would it make a difference to the people working there? Which story would you rather have appear in your local newspaper—that your hospital won JCAHO commendation or achieved Top 100 status?

The Top 100 Measures

In recent years a new annual report, *The 100 Top Hospitals: Benchmarks for Success,* produced jointly by HCIA, Inc. (HCIA) and William M. Mercer, Incorporated (Mercer), has added an interesting new dimension to identifying benchmark organizations in the industry. This approach develops a model of high performance for general acute care hospitals in the United States and identifies 100 of the top-performing hospitals on the basis of key measures related to clinical practices, operations, and financial management.[2] (Excluded from the study are children's, psychiatric, and rehabilitation hospitals, hospitals with fewer than twenty-five acute care beds or fewer than 500 total facility admissions, hospitals with a Medicare average length of stay greater than thirty days, and multilocation facilities filing consolidated Medicare cost report.)

The report attempts to establish industry benchmarks in the context of a rapidly changing health care industry and to recognize hospitals that demonstrate superior performance. Even though the measures used have been criticized for having evolved over the years, this seems to be a necessary problem of refinement in a dynamic and rapidly consolidating industry struggling to satisfy a demanding marketplace. Eight measures were used as of 1998, listed here in summary form (Morrissey, 1998d):

---

[2]I have borrowed from the 1994–1997 *Top 100 Hospitals,* published by HCIA-Mercer, in paraphrasing and in footnotes directly attributable to HCIA-Mercer writers. However, I have presented only those points of view which I felt fit the larger argument framed in this book. The curious reader will want to contact HCIA-Mercer on the Internet for the full content of their reports.

Clinical Practices

- Risk-adjusted mortality index. Number of actual deaths divided by the number expected, given the condition of each patient (a two-year sample).
- Risk-adjusted complications index. Number of actual complications divided by the number expected, given the condition of each patient admitted (a two-year sample).

Financial Management

- Expense per adjusted discharge. Total operating expenses divided by the number of discharges, adjusted for case mix and wages.
- Profitability (cash flow margin). The sum of net income, depreciation, and interest expense divided by the sum of net patient revenue and total other income.
- Productivity (total asset turnover ratio). Net patient revenue divided by total assets. Measures the amount of productivity a hospital achieves in relation to the assets it controls.

Operations

- Severity-adjusted average length of stay. Adjusted for differences in severity of illness.
- Proportion of outpatient revenue. Compare with total facility revenues.
- Index of total facility occupancy. Added in 1997, this is the sum of two measures: total occupancy rate during 1997, and the average of the percentage change in occupancy rate from 1996 to 1997 and from 1995 to 1996.

What makes the idea of pursuing Top 100 status as either an organizational goal or an industry report card is that it is based on objective, quantitative data that are consistent and complete across the United States. This methodology ensures that the focus is on statistical rather than anecdotal evidence for top performance. The HCIA-Mercer list allows a specific hospital to be compared against its peers if it is a general, short-term, acute care, non-federal U.S. hospital.

Peer Group Ranking

Each hospital in the resulting universe was assigned to one of five peer groups according to its location, number of beds in service, and teaching status. The five peer groups are hospitals with twenty-five to ninety-nine acute care beds, hospitals with 100–249 acute care beds, nonteaching hospitals (250 or more beds), teaching hospitals (250–399 beds), and major teaching hospitals (400 or more beds).

The eight performance-measure values for each hospital within each peer group are calculated with Medicare cost report and discharge data from the previous year. Within the peer groups, hospitals are ranked on the basis of their performance on each of the eight measures. Each hospital's performance-measure rankings are then summed to arrive at a total ranking for the hospital. The hospitals with the best total rankings in each peer group are selected as benchmark hospitals. The list of 100 top-performing hospitals includes a designated number of hospitals from each of the five groups.

Significant Findings

The results of the 100 Top Hospitals study demonstrate the continued improvement of the health care industry in the United States—the numbers are getting better. A number of findings from the period 1993–1998 are instructive.

• Benchmark hospitals continue to improve. The 100 top hospitals performed better than the previous year's list. Implication: Once a benchmark hospital leaves the starting gate in the journey to excellence, it may be increasingly difficult for competitors to catch up.

• Benchmark hospitals are plateauing. There is evidence that the early year gains of Top 100 hospitals in terms of cost cutting under managed care may be nearing an end. To move to the next higher level, the practice of medicine itself will have to be changed. Simple efficiencies in the old system will not yield enough gain for those who have largely implemented them; not cost cutting, but work process redesign and reconfiguration of services are the next steps.

- Winners tend to repeat and be consistent. In 1998, 63 percent of the top 100 had won the award at least once before. Winners tended to be institutions recognized as being well managed and producers of innovative and high-quality work but many were lesser-known facilities (that is, excellence is less a matter of reputation than determination). Each of the benchmark hospital groups exceeded the performances of their peer groups on all eight performance measures.[3] Implication: Effective managements get their organizations into a groove of winning, a habit borne out of orientation to goals, work, and measured performance.

- Five-year trends show a tougher playing field. Average length of stay and occupancy rates declined each year. The greatest decrease in length of stay was at teaching and major teaching hospitals (28 percent), whereas nonteaching hospitals had the greatest decrease in occupancy (13.4 percent over the five years). A second major finding was an increase of 22 percent in outpatient revenue. Implication: New services and settings signal the need for revamping the business.

- Managed care means less business for hospitals. It is not surprising that as the penetration of managed care increased, the average length of stay declined. In 1996, hospitals with a high penetration of managed care had a median average length of stay of 4.08 days versus 4.96 days for hospitals with a low penetration of managed care. High-penetration managed care settings were about 8 percent cheaper ($3,840) per adjusted discharge than the $4,170 charged in low-penetration hospitals. Low-penetration managed care hospitals derived 36.4 percent of business from outpatient services in 1996, whereas high-penetration managed care hospitals received only 29 percent, a finding largely due to payers having patients treated in nonhospital clinical settings. Implication: Operational Excellence as a management approach to

---

[3] In the HCIA-Mercer report writer's words, "Overall, the widest gaps between the benchmark hospitals and the peer groups can be seen in the financial measures of profitability, return on assets, and growth in equity. Furthermore, for all the hospital categories, the gap between the benchmark hospitals and their peer groups remains significantly wider for return on assets than profitability, suggesting that benchmarks are not only enjoying strong net income but are also, to an even greater extent, redeploying unproductive assets."

market reality fits the managed care environment, as do nonhospital care settings.

• Benchmark hospitals may be favored by geography. The geographic concentration of benchmark hospitals seems to correlate with the South, which represents 43 percent of all benchmark hospitals (the West has 18 percent). One hypothesis put forward by the Mercer researchers is that greater competition, driven by investor-owned and for-profit hospitals, may be driving these regions up the performance curve (Internet documents from HCIA-Mercer, "Implications of the Benchmark Study," 1994, 1995, 1997).[4] Although competition is an anathema to some, it has the potential to increase organizational strength. Implication: Leaders who want their organizations to be excellent also want strong competitors.

Implications for Other Hospitals

Among the more challenging implications of the standardization concept is this: If all U.S. acute care hospitals were to perform at the level of the 100 benchmark hospitals, the results for the industry and the nation would be dramatic. According to statements by HCIA-Mercer (1994, 1995, 1997; "100 Top Hospitals Studies," 1994–1998):

• Average lengths of stay for complex cases at the Top 100 are 7 percent shorter, occupancy is 22 percent higher, and employment of staff members per unit is 18 percent lower.
• Inpatient mortality and complications are 22 percent lower.

---

[4]In the HCIA-Mercer researcher's words, "The superior performance of hospitals in the South, as well as the significant proportion of benchmark hospitals located there, can in part be explained by the fact that the South has been relatively free of regulation and has been targeted by investor-owned facilities seeking to gain regional market footholds. Investor-owned chains with facilities located in this region are giving not-for-profit hospitals a serious competitive challenge not only financially, but clinically as well." The report further hypothesizes that the paucity of benchmark hospitals in the Northeast may be caused by an overly regulated environment.

- Top 100 Hospitals are 38 percent more profitable, and growth in equity and return on assets are significantly higher.
- Quality (measured by complications and mortality) is 16 percent better than at other hospitals.
- If the nation's hospitals operated at the Top 100 benchmarks, expenses would be reduced an aggregate of $26.3 billion a year, and charges would be reduced an aggregate of $43 billion per year.

The unanswered question raised in such a report is what causes this success. Successful results are nearly always obtainable when best practice processes are used. An organization's success is assured when it correctly manages clinical and nonclinical work, focuses with intensity on Customer needs, builds an empowered workforce, and runs on the high octane of a superior culture. That is clearly demonstrated in the case of the Top 100. These results didn't just magically appear, nor were they a statistical fluke. They were created by aggressive management teams.

There are clearly winners and losers in the American hospital industry, and the nation can't afford the losers anymore. Leaders must decide whether the Top 100 is worth pursuing. If others have done it, would your team want to do it, too? I don't believe that the Top 100 criteria are the only or best measures an organization might want to strive for, but they are a starting point, one that can be used by "take it to 'em" leaders as a challenge to their own organization. Some observers note that there can be problems with Top 100 Hospitals criteria (Weissenstein and Moore, 1998). Some have suggested that it is possible to manipulate numbers in one year to produce positive statistics. Others tell stories of incidents of horrible care in some of the winners. So although the measured dimensions are impressive, lots of problems may remain. The best course may be to understand that achieving Top 100 status is not necessarily a desirable or a final goal. A review panel of executives consulted in writing this book chose to accept five of the Top 100 eight performance measures to include in their list of stretch goals and balanced scorecard approaches (Chapter Two). Their thinking was to use at least parts of the Top 100 list as an approach to move things forward and galvanize people's thinking.

A Proposal to Raise Standards

From a management perspective, and ignoring the real political world that has managed to induce health care into a coma, might there be an easier, cleaner, more sensible way to use standards to further the nation's health? Would it also be advantageous to set out a simple set of elements that would govern all providers, making their compliance duties much clearer and removing the ambiguity that plagues the industry? The following outline would be closer to what payers and consumers would probably prefer. It has the profoundly important benefit of making life easier for providers and practitioners.

1. Establish a national set of mandatory standards that all providers must meet, with detailed specifications for each type of service provided. Each professional group would have input to this process. The industry can no longer remain a collection of cottages or separate professional fiefdoms, but must mature to benchmark levels as have other industries. Standards would not be minimal—the convoy mentality of gearing speed to the slowest ship won't do. Standards levels should be set at current best practices, or as close to them as the political process will allow.

2. Each profession would produce endorsed best practice protocols and either directly or under sponsorship be responsible to upgrade these through normal channels of research and innovation by providers. Best practices would be considered the performance floor, but provider improvements beyond this level would be sought to gain competitive advantage.

3. Establish a similar consensus of measures to be used. More than one vendor could be used to process and manage the data, but all would use standardized formats and content. The databases currently being built will need to be coordinated and standardized, but represent a substantial and helpful asset for change.

4. Quarterly updates to the list of standards, protocols, and measures would be published instead of the continuous, uncoordinated, poorly communicated stream now used. An example can be found in software companies that provide quarterly or semiannual software updates on the Internet. Sufficient schedules and structured guidelines for implementation would be provided.

This continuous upgrading challenge might require the assistance of consultants (and thereby provide an opportunity for free enterprise).

5. Beef up an enforcement arm—some combination of state and federal government—to conduct audits and administer sanctions. This would be an extension of what is now done, with full public disclosure of each provider's state of compliance with standards. Enforcement is a legitimate role of government in protecting the public interest, and accreditation is never going to be effective as enforcement (accreditation would cease as a process and expense). The public and payers will administer economic punishment to poor providers as part of a normal free market function, either by closing them down or motivating them to improve.

6. In line with these proposals, legislatures would provide tort reform to protect hospitals and health practitioners as long as they followed best practice protocols. Providers not using best practices would be left open to prosecution, for here at last would be the ultimate lawyer's argument against malpractice.

From a management perspective, this simple logic is what is needed. Although a lot of debate would be required to get past the "ifs, ands, and buts," it's a logic that would vastly improve on today's less than best practices.

Who wins under this approach? Everybody wins. Associations and their member professionals have a strong hand in determining how their profession should be practiced. Provider organizations have a clear structure to follow rather than the current quagmire of conflict they experience. Government fulfills its responsibility to the public without interfering in setting standards that should be determined by others. Payers win because best practices equate to higher quality, best cost, and far happier patients. An organization's Associates win because pride in performance is possible only when work is done at best levels. Most important of all, patients and their families win, and they win big.

What would it take for this logic to become a framework for recrafting the national approach to health care standards and implementation? Association leaders might have some ideas for joint conferences to establish consensus. Legislators could provide a law that calls for the implementation of such an agenda while allowing involved parties to fill in the details as to how to sculpt each part.

What's the alternative? Another twenty years of continuous bickering, or working on this piece or that piece of the problem? Do we really want to build the house this way, or are we at a point that we ought to agree on a blueprint of what the place is going to look like?

Advice to Provider and Payer Managements

If the current confused standards environment does not move forward, and outsiders (government, associations, researchers) are ineffectual, the best course for management is to aggressively move the organization upward regardless. It is more difficult and far more expensive to have to do this without a national consensus on standards, but it would be the second best course.

Payers can serve their own and beneficiaries' interests most by encouraging selected providers to push the standards button. By partnering on implementing best practices (or incentivizing or cheerleading), payers can be an effective driver of change. Payers should also consider involving employers and business coalitions to help drive this effort. From the standpoint of the bill-paying parties, direct involvement in this manner is the surest short-term strategy. If development of standards is insufficient by others along the lines I have suggested, it may prove to be the only long-term, workable strategy to get costs and quality under control while simultaneously increasing payer's customer retention, a retention driven by satisfaction with provider services.

Conclusion

Health care standards are in a state of flux. Older definitions, concepts, and levels of performance are rapidly being eclipsed by the push for data-based measurement. Alert managements, along with consumers and payers, will continue to push performance gains that represent measurably valid improvements in care. We now have a major opportunity to gain the high ground quickly in competitive situations or to get the internal organization aligned around the concept of really elevating what we do. In the next chapter we'll look at an extended case study of McDonald's, an organization that has followed the dictates of Operational Excellence and strategic standardization, to see what parallels might be drawn in restructuring health care organizations.

Work-Out Session

1. If your organization currently subscribes to JCAHO accreditation, is it done primarily to gain reimbursement or are these standards truly seen as elevating care in your organization? What could be done to make these standards of greater benefit to the organization?

2. Would pursuit of Top 100 status, or some other national standing such as the 95th percentile on Customer satisfaction, add something to the verve and energy of your shop?

3. Which describes the view of your organization: There is resistance or passive compliance to existing standards; or there is active pursuit of performance levels beyond the regulators. What are the implications of your answer?

4. The management of quality is an internal management responsibility. In group discussion, identify where your organization is in need of tighter or renewed discipline. What priorities for action emerge from this list?

5. Has the organization fallen into the trap of assigning quality to a staff unit or committee instead of seeing it as an integral responsibility of all areas? How can this be corrected?

6. Where would better measurement, and communication of the findings to all staff, be a positive prescription?

7. Has quality of technical services and interpersonal interaction become core to the culture, or is it something that seems just pasted on? (Assume that people do care and are committed — what's missing from the execution of quality, what's deficient in work procedures and training?)

Part Three

Commonsense Solutions for Uncommon Performance

*There is in the worst of fortune
The best chances for a happy change.*
—EURIPIDES

There is a time for talking and debate and a time for action. Cutting through the intricacies of the health care system requires a commitment to turning ideas into reality, the hard work of attacking problems, and the weapons of new techniques and old-fashioned common sense. In this part of the book we'll examine a number of techniques that, taken together, can greatly assist the work of changing how our organizations perform.

The good news is that we have no shortage of answers to problems. The difficulty is in taking advantage of them, for we must first radically alter the work relationship and cut a new deal with the health care team.

Chapter Five

Moving to McDonaldland

Hospitals are moving toward a future of standardized health care. This will mean consistent quality delivery and lower cost. This chapter will show what standardization can mean to organizational business performance. The clarity and sureness of such a future can be of immense benefit in the rocky and fragmented world of nonstandardized health care today. A standardized future need not be threatening, and its creation can be one of health care management's finest acts.

This chapter provides a case example of Operational Excellence in action, McDonald's, where success is derived in large part from standardization. As an organization, McDonald's is a part of American culture. For instance:

A truck driver stopped at a McDonald's for lunch. He ordered a cheeseburger, fries, and a coffee. As he was about to eat, three motorcycles pulled up outside. The bikers came in, and one grabbed the trucker's cheeseburger and took a bite from it. The second one drank the trucker's coffee, and the third wolfed down the fries.

The truck driver didn't say a word. He simply got up and left. When he was gone, one of the motorcyclists said, "He ain't much of a man, is he?" "He's not much of a driver, either," the cashier replied. "He just backed his truck over three motorcycles."

McDonald's competitors, no doubt, often feel run over as well. This worldwide fast food chain represents in many ways what the hospital industry must become and illustrates many of the central prescriptions of this book. As a case study, there are obvious limitations. Running a hamburger stand is not the same as running a health care business. But in this relatively simple business are found a number of powerful ideas that can benefit your organization. This industry leader

- Follows a clearly defined Operational Excellence strategy positioned distinctly in the market in terms of providing exactly what their customers want—good-quality, affordable food, with no hassles, and fast.
- Provides breakthrough benchmarking, even though it originally copied best practices elsewhere—whether or not you like the product, nobody runs a hamburger stand better.
- Standardizes operations around the globe, allowing regional menu differences where dictated by the market, but remaining standardized within the region.
- Achieves unfailing control over quality and cost.

McDonald's is the largest and best-known global food service retailer. With over 14,000 stands in the United States and a total of over 23,000 in 109 countries worldwide, it employs nearly a million people and accounts for more than seven cents out of every dollar that Americans spend on food outside the home. The average American lives within four minutes of a virtually ubiquitous McDonald's stand, the single largest feeder of people on planet earth. McDonald's serves over thirty million people daily, over eighteen million of them in the United States. With annual 1998 sales of $8.2 billion, a sales growth rate of 9 percent, a market capitalization of $45 billion, and a compound annual total return of 17 percent over the past ten years, McDonald's is the only company in the Standard & Poor's 500 to have publicly reported more than 120 consecutive quarters of year-to-year combined increases in revenues, income, and earnings per share since 1965. *Better Investing* ranked McDonald's as the most widely held common stock by individuals and investment clubs. This hasn't been a bad stock to own. Their vision statement contains their view of how the company intends to implement Operational Excellence. McDonald's clearly understands the standards issue: "Our Vision: McDonald's vision is to dominate the global food service industry. Global dominance means setting the performance standard for customer satisfaction and increasing market share and profitability through successfully implementing our Convenience, Value, and Execution Strategies" (McDonald's website).

What do you think of McDonald's? It's doubtful anyone would say they've never tasted a better hamburger, or that their stands are the best restaurants in America. But what it has achieved is a winning combination of good enough food, at a good enough price, available anywhere you want it on the planet, with a playroom to park the kids, and all this done *fast*.

Part of what McDonald's provides is what it doesn't give you: Whereas other fast food providers get more publicity than they want in terms of food poisoning incidents, this never seems to be the case at McDonald's. As an organization it has converted the lowly hamburger stand into an international symbol of excellence, making it one of the most widely studied organizations in the world. Say what you will, the market judgment is that this organization, three times as large and many times more successful than its closest rival, Burger King, is the provider of choice. Indeed, the organization's occasional errors (like the 1996 disappointing results from the Arch Deluxe) are widely discussed because it is so unusual for this machine-like organization to stumble.

As metaphor, McDonald's approach to management, not the business it's in, suggests a number of positive avenues for health care management to pursue. Should we run our health care organization like a hamburger stand? No, but maybe you ought to run your business the way McDonald's runs its business.

McDonald's own analysis of why it has done well is that it sticks to the basics and keeps everything simple. According to Shelby Yastrow, senior VP, these are the guidelines that underlie its success (as cited in Edmund, 1990):

- Stick to what you do best. McDonald's has resisted diversification, service expansion, and acquisitions. Though the company has a hotel for visitors and students at Hamburger University in Oak Brook, Illinois, it's run by Hyatt. Although it buys and sells more real estate than any company in the world, it uses outside realtors. Prescription health care implication: Focus on the core businesses, outsource where possible, cut back on peripheral activities.

- Sweat the small stuff. Handle details well to keep big problems from developing. "Ninety-nine percent of our success depends on what happens in that last three feet of counter separating us from our customer. That's where we focus our thinking."

Prescription health care implication: Start at the "last three feet" —the interaction points with Customers—for instance, admitting, bedside interactions, the moment they open their bill. Work back from there to find out what details need fixing.

- Everybody knows the business. No new staffer, secretary, or attorney can start a job at McDonald's until they've worked in a stand, serving the food, cleaning up. Every year all employees, including management and officers, must spend time again seeing the business where it really happens. Prescription health care implication: Get executives out of their offices, make them work in the departments they supervise. Give all new hires at least a short stint in a nursing unit. One result: A reduction in remote control management and interdepartmental tensions.

- Get rid of bureaucracy. Organizational charts and standing committees are at a minimum at McDonald's, and little time is spent on written reports. Communicate whenever possible by direct talking. Make every decision at the lowest possible level, including annual budgets, expenditures, and hiring. Prescription health care implication: Start by asking managers what policies restrict their ability to get action. Hospitals are so worried about making mistakes that they don't make enough progress. Mistakes cannot be controlled by writing another memo.

- Understand the difference between planning and preparing. "Planning is thinking, preparing is doing." If it works, do more. If it doesn't work, change it. Prescription health care implication: Too much planning in health care, not enough doing. Adjust the focus. Things aren't working; try something different.

- Achievement comes from risk. According to senior VP Yastrow, "I've never seen anybody held back for taking a chance or making a mistake, but I have seen people's careers sidetracked because they couldn't make a decision or because they played it safe." Prescription health care implication: Create a culture in which people don't feel subservient, subordinate, or passive aggressive. The residue of old management in the health care industry is often manifested in passive managers and low morale. Until that's changed, business performance won't improve.

Why can't Burger King beat McDonald's (or K Mart beat Wal-Mart, or Universal beat Disney, or United Express beat Southwest)? Trying to understand why an industry's number two can't overtake the leader is a fascinating area of study. You can walk into McDonald's and see what it does. Hundreds of articles, books, and case studies have been written on the company. Why can't their success be duplicated?

Although the answer has a lot of specific details, the overriding issues are standards and culture. The following are examples of McDonald's approach to achieving Operational Excellence (Peters, 1995):

- Whereas national competitors typically have three to eight service systems, McDonald's has only one on which all improvement efforts have been concentrated.
- Although competitors still use squeeze bottles to apply mustard and ketchup, McDonald's has specially made dispensers that put on all condiments in a five-point star pattern with a single squeeze, thus saving seconds. Seconds add up when you repeat the process 100 billion times.
- Instead of innovating by providing get-it-yourself drinks (à la Burger King), McDonald's created a two-window drive-through to speed up the process and avoid having unsanitary money handled by the people handling food orders.
- Like General Electric, McDonald's did away with their strategic planning unit. They practice SCR (strategic customer response) instead. By intensely monitoring Customers' opinions, they move rapidly whenever those opinions change, as when Customers suggested they use recycled materials instead of plastic foam materials (savings of 7 cents per container). What's the strategy? Simple. When Customers want something different, respond.

A Detail-Controlling System

Control of detail is a central management issue. Consider the lowly French fry. It's not a big deal to make one, just slice a spud and fry it. But in the McDonald's system, it becomes a highly unique item, with specially designed work processes and technology to produce it. The McDonald's French fry points the way to what American health care must do if it is to achieve its rightful place in the future. It is the epitome of standardization, and it exemplifies a thorough systems approach and a fanatical management philosophy.

Of course running a health care system is not comparable to running a hamburger stand. Cooking fries is an easy job compared to the infinitely more difficult tasks of patient care. But surely the more important work of patient care deserves just as much diligence as McDonald's devotes to the French fry (Love, 1995):

• Demand. Cook 3000 pounds of potatoes/stand weekly at 23,000 stands worldwide. All batches must be identical in look, taste, water content, crispness. No variation in the final product is allowed, for customers want "unfailing quality."

• Spud. Based entirely on exhaustive customer research on taste preferences and other expectations, the specifications are

Species must be No. 1 Idaho Russet

Width, 9/32″

Color, a specific Pantone number, not lighter, not darker

Harvested potatoes must have a solids content of 21 percent, not
   more, not less

• Suppliers. Farmers must produce a potato that meets specifications on shape, uniformity, moisture, starch, and sugar. McDonald's has outsourced all foodstuffs, and thus made a number of growers and processors wealthy. Planting and fertilizing procedures must be followed exactly by all growers. Each must use identical storage equipment set at identical temperature and humidity levels. If a supplier produces any variation from McDonald's specifications, that supplier is out. McDonald's doesn't foster a punitive relationship with its suppliers; it is just a demanding customer. McDonald's is universally well thought of by its suppliers. But as an organization running a service business, McDonald's knows that quality must be controlled at its source upstream in the supply chain. Should health care suppliers be more tightly controlled by specific standards and a narrower range of supplies and supplier organizations?

• Equipment. Fries are cooked in a two-stage process: first blanched and then cooked at the moment of demand. Special

McDonald's-designed cookers hold the cooking oil temperature to within one degree of the ideal starting temperature. The cooking oil (the same special blend used by all stands worldwide) must then rise precisely three degrees by the end of the cook cycle, which is exactly two minutes and fifty seconds, with a rapid return to starting temperature for the next cooking cycle. This is accomplished by automated temperature control, since it proved impossible for humans to control temperature manually. Each batch is shaken at twenty seconds with a beeper reminder. Cooked fries can be kept in a finished hopper for seven minutes and then must be tossed out if not sold. Is there a need to standardize the technology in use in health care?

• Culture. Key to ▓▓▓ organization's success is a culture that lets Associates know how they're doing through rigorous review and rewards, and gives them the pride of achievement through systematic training and internal promotion. Perhaps McDonald's can't offer a wide range of jobs, but they make the most out of what they have. Whether it's the All-American Marching Band or Ronald McDonald, the culture works to have fun at work—a helpful prescription for many health care organizations. Said McDonald's first franchisee: "All the advertising, all the gimmicks, all of the new menu items just won't do. It's the day-to-day attention to operations that does it. Well-trained employees, who have an interest and pride in their work, keep the business on a one-to-one basis, between customer and employee." Do health care workers have as much fun and pride? Are they trained as well?

• Results. One could describe the results in terms of market share or profitability, but let's be more personal. Over all the years of experience you've had with McDonald's, did you ever fail to get the fries you ordered? Were they ever not up to the standard? I've asked that question in a number of health care groups and it's rare that even a single hand will go up. Now consider these questions. In just the last ninety days, have you asked for information or ordered items within your organization and not been able to get what you needed, when you needed them? Have you ever been dissatisfied with what you received? The response I typically get in a group setting is over half the group raises their hands. For fun, try this sampling of your system's response capability at your next management meeting.

What is seen in the French fry example is extreme attention to detail in a refined process that took years to develop as a best practice. It is precisely that focus that is needed now in defining best practices and then standardizing them in health care. What is called for is the application of management to each and every necessary task in health care.

Review of Standards

There is another element of McDonald's fries worth noting, for it directly bears on hospital standards. In the United States, McDonald's has an army of 400 service "consultants" with a checklist of over 500 items. They help to keep everyone on their toes through the many unannounced visits made to each stand each year. Items being audited include bathroom cleanliness, staff performance, parking lot appearance, customer service, and even whether open cardboard boxes of items in storage have had their flaps trimmed off. Added to these on-site checklist inspections are statistics on turnover, register errors, and other items needing attention (which are then used in other, more detailed store audits). To add teeth to the surprise inspections, failure to pass any of them can result in loss of the owner's franchise. There is no fooling around in this tough system that has made a majority of its owners millionaires. This inspection system definitely does not resemble the once-every-three-years scheduled JCAHO visit. The contrast is stark. By comparison, health care is woefully inattentive to its business. It is doubtful whether many accredited hospitals could pass a McDonald's field audit.

Training a Million-Person Workforce

Did you ever try to manage one teenager at home? Try managing several hundred thousand of them, just one of McDonald's challenges. Lots of things go into the leadership of people: selection, recognition, compensation, achievement opportunity. And certainly training. How does McDonald's, as one of the world's largest employers, train so many people, many of them part-timers, and train them quickly so they can be productive?

One of the key factors is the intensive training given to each restaurant manager and the two levels of supervisors that report to him. Some of this is done at Hamburger University, much of it is done in the store, all of it is tightly scripted and standardized.

Hamburger University provides the extensive course work needed for franchisees and managers to earn their required B.S. and M.S. certificates in Hamburgerology. (All management training is done at Hamburger University to keep content standard.)

In each restaurant there is a crew room, where training videos and manuals are used in following a prescribed curriculum. Training is consistent worldwide. Trainees are walked through classroom and on-the-job training in a rigorous approach that efficiently converts even high school dropouts to well-functioning staff in a matter of weeks. Training is clearly one of McDonald's greatest competitive weapons. Their training videotapes send the exact words (in any language) and pictures needed to show how each task should be done. Training also includes a task list for each job, a curriculum guide that specifies sequence, duration, and repetitions needed for each task's mastery, and a checkoff list as steps are completed. Each staffer keeps her own training log, completion of which qualifies for pay increases.

Compare this simple but thorough approach to how a majority of hourly health workers encounter their employment situation. They receive inadequate orientation, they aren't checked out on the tasks they're being paid to do, and they're supervised by managers with little leadership training. McDonald's averages thirty-five hours of annual training per hire, whereas one estimate is that hospitals average six hours per person.

Could Your Suppliers Meet McDonald's Standards?

Quality begins upstream, as any fan of continuous improvement knows. If problems are solved at the supplier end, or in the department handling the patient previous to yours, those problems don't have to be revisited when the work moves to you. Here is a brief illustration of the control that McDonald's has over its suppliers, an alliance that produces success for all parties, and a model that hospitals need to imitate.

History. Founded in 1958, the HAVI Corporation has only one customer—McDonald's (HAVI is not allowed other customers). The company acts as the sole distributor for all items used in an eleven-state midwestern region. As the only source for the 3,300 McDonald's restaurants in this area, HAVI must maintain contacts with all manufacturers of baked goods, paper products, machinery, store fixtures, and so forth and maintain sufficient inventory to service their customer. The company operates out of three distribution centers with a fleet of trucks assigned to subregions.

Operating environment. This unusual arrangement came about as a result of a strategic decision made by McDonald's that they are in the fast food service business, not the distribution business. A high control organization, McDonald's sets tough product specifications on all its suppliers and quickly replaces any supplier who does not maintain standards. There has been virtually no supplier turnover in decades because suppliers manage as excellently as their giant Customer.

The relationship with HAVI was established on a handshake agreement between McDonald's president Ray Kroc and HAVI president Bob Rocque. There is no written contract between the two organizations. McDonald's maintains control over HAVI by setting standards; for example, all delivery trucks must be steam cleaned daily (trucks cleaner than many of those delivering hospital supplies).

Standards with an impact. Then there's the 95–95 standard. Ninety-five percent of the items that a store manager orders must be delivered within one week, the balance within two weeks; 95 percent of all deliveries must be within specified delivery hours, a just-in-time (JIT) model (no trucks are to be in the lots during meal times). Meeting the 95–95 standard creates tremendous logistics and inventory problems and puts HAVI in the difficult role of having to iron out any problems with dozens of suppliers, who first have to get their items to HAVI warehouses.

The bottom line in the relationship between these two organizations is that subsequent to any week that HAVI fails to meet either of the 95 percent standards, the company has only one week to get back to standard. Failure to correct means that McDonald's would look for a distributor to replace HAVI. The stakes represent a choice between a multimillion dollar bottom line or instant financial ruin.

In front of each of the distribution centers are three flag poles flying the American, McDonald's, and HAVI flags. In any week in which 95–95 is not met, the HAVI flag is lowered to half mast. On Monday mornings, employees entering the parking lot see the lowered flag and report immediately to their supervisor for consultation and problem solving. On these occasions employees are seen running into the building to get to their department conferences.

Values centered managing. To further clarify his direction to the organization, Bob Rocque has clarified the key values that staff are to follow at all times. These are their principal accountabilities, listed in priority sequence—and all must be accomplished. Hourly Associates' prime values are the 4 Ss; all members of management follow the 5 Ps (see below):

Values as Shorthand Direction

Associate Values	Management Values
Service	People
Safety	Philosophy
Sanitation	Policy
Security	Procedure
	Profitability

The 4 Ss and 5 Ps are clarified and defined in operational terms and form the basis for self-governance and self-management. The organization has never missed the 95–95 standard more than a week in a row.

Health Care Suppliers Face a New Future

A shakeout in health care suppliers can be expected, both in their numbers and in how they operate with their provider Customers. Strategic standardization means the implementation of a number of important principles:

• Reduce the number of suppliers. As reported in the *Chicago Tribune,* as Chrysler's revitalized organization continues to gather speed, it has reduced the number of its primary or "first-tier" suppliers from 1200 to 150 ("Chrysler Will Reduce Number of Suppliers," 1995). This saves not only money because of more massive purchasing power and lower distribution costs for the supplier, but also saves time through simplification at the provider's purchasing site. It also allows providers, or their purchasing groups, to work more closely with suppliers in creating better systems. Part of the reduction in numbers among suppliers will come from competition to fit into this new relationship. Although this process is well along in terms of materials purchasing, the shakeout among other areas such as consultant usage or information services has proceeded more slowly.

• Reduce the number of supply varieties. In Chrysler's case, the numbers of fasteners used in assembling a car dropped from eighty-seven to nine and the number of tools to apply them from thirty-six to three. Think of the gains in training simplification alone. Many hospitals have been making substantial progress on this front, and it is also supportive in installing clinical protocols.

• Give end users final decision. Tenet Health Care has established a successful model of letting physicians and nurses make the final call on some supply contracts. Purchasing submits a list of vendors allowed to compete and handles final contract negotiations. Clinicians then evaluate bids based on clinical preference and companies' reputations. The financial people pledged to abstain from influencing the decision, so the lowest cost bidder does not always win. But the company nevertheless saves money by gaining internal compliance and by awarding sole contractor status (Hensley, 1997).

• Set product and service standards high in the process. Remember Deming's advice to buy the best tools, don't just go for the deal of the week (Deming, 1986). Best practices require best tools and best supplies, which sometimes cost more initially. The evidence is that they cost far less in the long run because of fewer breakdowns, interchangeability, training support, and other contributing elements.

• Look for efficient consumer response. Savvy suppliers are utilizing principles pioneered in the grocery industry that are known as *efficient consumer response*. Elements include bar coding with UPNs (universal product numbers), EDI (electronic data interchange) so products can be bought electronically, continuous replenishment to speed stocking and keep inventories low, and ABC (activity-based costing) to account for the cost of services (Scott, 1996). New EDI standards set by the government are expected to save $42.3 billion over six years in claims handling costs alone, based in part on Arizona providers' experiences (Moore, 1996).

• Pick suppliers as lifetime partners. High standards also apply to the quality of the people and their organizations who will act as your suppliers. Pick those you are willing to work with for decades. This is a partnership—each partner wins only when they are looking out for the other's interests. McDonald's puts high demands on suppliers but gives them a tremendous amount of business and sustains long-term relationships. Suppliers should not be considered throw-away members of the team.

• Set goals for suppliers. Use the BHAG concept externally, not just for challenging internal operations. Chrysler, who has the best relations with suppliers of any Big Three car maker, requests suppliers to save them 5 percent overall each year on the parts they buy, and also comes up with ideas for specific parts they want made for less (their remote-control keyfob costs $3 less than Ford's). They've even coached suppliers to tear Chrysler's competitors' cars apart to figure out how they're built and apply those ideas to Chrysler (benchmarking).

Building a world-class health care organization also requires building a world-class supply chain. That supply chain begins with external suppliers but continues in-house. Apply these same principles there. A practice we've seen success with has been to have nursing units rate departments who act as their internal suppliers. The focus is on finding things to improve, not people to punish. Improved supply solutions from dietary, lab, or admitting departments, for example, then win awards from their Customer units.

The Argument for Focused Factories

McDonald's succeeds in part because it tries to do a few things well. Along similar lines, Regina Herzlinger's excellent book, *Market Driven Health Care* (1997), argues for standardization of health care procedures and proposes that hospitals accomplish this by concentrating on a shorter list of diagnostic categories rather than trying to be all things to all people.

In manufacturing, this argument dates back to a 1974 *Harvard Business Review* article, "The Focused Factory," which provided a series of prescriptions that proved beneficial as American factories revitalized in the 1980s. The author, Wickham Skinner, pointed out that factories that were overly complex—because of too many product lines and product variations—were at the heart of America's productivity crisis (Skinner, 1974):

> A factory that focuses on a narrow product mix for a particular market niche will outperform the conventional plant, which attempts a broader mission. Because its equipment, supporting systems, and procedures can concentrate on a limited task for one set of customers, its costs . . . are likely to be lower than a conventional plant. But, more important, such a plant can become a competitive weapon because its entire apparatus is focused to accomplish the . . . task . . . demanded by the company's overall strategy. . . .
>
> Focused manufacturing plants are surprisingly rare. Instead, the conventional factory produces many products for numerous customers in a variety of markets, thereby demanding the performance of a multiplicity of manufacturing tasks all at once from one set of assets and people. Its rationale is "economy of scale" and lower capital investment. . . . However, the result, more often than not, is a hodgepodge of compromises, a high overhead, a[n] . . . organization that is constantly in hot water with customers.

Compare Skinner's comments to the warning noted earlier to avoid "dabbling" in terms of market positioning, a lesson mastered by market leaders. Skinner recommends that producers focus each plant on a short list of products, technologies, and markets; structure basic policies, procedures, and support services on one explicit production objective instead of many inconsistent, conflicting, and implicit objectives; see the problem as being one that affected the efficiency of the entire organization, not just the efficiency of the work force.

Herzlinger's idea is that such principles would also apply in health care. Other work suggests that the average complexity of the American hospital is twenty times that of the average factory—an indication of over-complexity and accidents in the making. Health care will always be a more complex process than running a factory or a hamburger stand, but its present Rube Goldberg systems are drastically in need of simplification. This argument is supported by numerous studies showing that quality is directly tied to volume. An editorial in *Modern Healthcare* put it this way ("For Good Outcomes, More Is Better," 1997): "The growing use of benchmarking and measurement of medical outcomes usually leads to the same conclusion: The more often a hospital or physician performs a procedure, the higher the success rate. The latest evidence comes from an HHS [Health and Human Services] report highlighting the strides achieved in organ transplantation. More transplant surgeries are completed without a hitch and recipients are living longer. The heavy-volume transplant programs are by far the most successful."

The reasons this occurs are numerous: The experience of physicians and staff has led to improved skills, best equipment, better access to and use of current state-of-the-art knowledge, and more established work protocols with supporting departments. The evidence clearly leads one to conclude that adding new services to stay competitive should be avoided if volumes will be low.

Simplify, Now

Even though it may not be possible to retrofit many of America's hospitals immediately in terms of facility layout or range of services, it is still possible to

- Enter negotiations with other providers to trade one service line for another to build volume and move toward focused factory status.
- Outsource as many functions as possible. This allows the organization to focus on its primary objectives. Another plus is that a standardized best practice model is typically what contractors are able to supply; Marriott exemplifies this.
- Standardize purchases for pharmacy, materials, and technology. The minimal goal should be to at least reduce the number of options to a manageable list. One side benefit is lower costs in exchange for greater volume given to fewer suppliers.
- Find and eliminate excess work: Unnecessary reports, meetings, and authorizations typically constitute 30 percent of all work done by managers.
- Define and streamline all existing procedures. On noncritical, nonclinical procedures, a less-than-best practice will usually

get better results than a perfect one *if* it is faster and simpler to use. Here the tradeoff favors speed over perfection. Striving for perfection on nonessentials is a trap to avoid.

- Improve all key procedures to best-practice levels, particularly those identified as high cost, high volume, or high risk or as having high variance of outcome.
- Automate as many core and high-volume tasks as possible.
- Upgrade human resource practices, particularly selection and training, and institute more open job design.

These elements, all part of future high-performance health care, can be put in place now to obtain benefits.

Conclusion

McDonald's is a clear example of an organization successfully pursuing an Operational Excellence strategy. To carry it out, they defined tough standards and then standardized operations to those of best practices. In keeping control of operations, they begin upstream with suppliers. They never assume that everything's OK but aggressively keep monitoring the system through a balance of data and on-site eyeballing. They work a lot on culture and pride, knowing that ultimately that drives the business.

This chapter has illustrated how these same principles may be used by health care to make major improvements. In the next chapter we'll examine the difficult problem of how to create a new organization capable of delivering best practices by completely redesigning the work environment and upgrading the culture. We'll look at how to build a new organization that can deliver the kind of outcomes required by the new environment. This new organization—the New American Hospital—mimics the best management practices found in benchmark organizations.

Work-Out Session

1. Where does the McDonaldland metaphor work in thinking about how to better manage your health care organization? Where does the metaphor break down?
2. Compare the methods at your shop with McDonald's to see where more work needs to be done in your shop: controlling

suppliers upstream, tough standards and defined procedures, product specs that match customer expectations, better tools, consistent and intensive training.

3. What kinds of work and controls do managers find themselves doing in health care organizations that don't match the above list? Where are work habits and procedures off-base in not meeting these criteria?

4. In the HAVI case, management practices values-centered management (know and live the values rather than merely supervise) and visual feedback on group performance. Might this approach work in your organization? Would it be an easier and more effective way to control performance?

5. What other management elements are at work in the McDonald's organization that are not mentioned in the chapter? Would they provide needed functions in your shop?

Chapter Six

Creating a New American Hospital

Coaches live or die on their win/loss record. If the team wins, fans name their babies after them. If the team loses. . . . During a bad stretch when Lou Holtz was football coach at Arkansas, he once opened his weekly TV program with, "Welcome to the Lou Holtz Show. Unfortunately, I'm Lou Holtz!"

It's the same in management. We want our team to win. The team requires the kind of supportive organization that will allow it to win. What kind of health care organization will it take to deliver performances that meet the ever higher standards the market demands? It's possible to build all kinds of organizations, but most would not be able to deliver what the market calls for in terms of quality, cost, and Customer satisfaction. Detroit wouldn't build a two-seat sports car if the objective was to create a truck. What should a health care organization look like if it is expected to produce superior results? How should it be structured and equipped? How would jobs be designed? What should leaders do to run it right? This chapter describes a new American health care organization that has the capability to turn out better quality at lower cost and with happier Customers and more motivated staff.

It's one thing to say that health care should pursue the standardization of best practices, but without some organizing principles, some conceptual architecture, we might have a mishmash of great practices without a cohesive whole. What should the "big picture" be that will form an overall scheme of organization? Best practices are like having a thousand jigsaw puzzle pieces. We need the cover picture of the jigsaw puzzle box as a model to put them together.

Stealing from the Best

In 1993 I published an account of our then ten-year experience in installing an organizational development model termed the *New American Hospital* (Sherman, 1993). The concept was to install as many best practices from benchmark companies as possible, adapt them to the special case of the hospital, and see whether they worked. As an example, notice how different the picture of Wal-Mart, a low-cost provider, is from the way many hospitals are being run. The following ideas are excerpted from Sam Walton's book, *Sam Walton: Made in America* (Walton and Huey, 1992).

Sam Walton's Rules for Business Building

- Rule 1: *Commit* to your business. Believe in it more than anybody else. I think I overcame every single one of my personal short-comings by the sheer passion I brought to my work. I don't know if you're born with this kind of passion or if you can learn it. But I do know you need it. If you love your work, you'll be out there every day trying to do it the best you possibly can, and pretty soon everybody around will catch the passion from you—like a fever.

- Rule 2: *Share* your profits with all your Associates, and treat them as partners. In turn they will treat you as a partner, and together you will all perform beyond your wildest expectations. Remain a corporation and retain control if you like, but behave as a servant leader in a partnership. Encourage your Associates to hold a stake in the company. Offer discounted stock, and grant them stock for their retirement. It's the single best thing we ever did.

- Rule 3: *Motivate* your partners. Money and ownership alone aren't enough. Constantly, day by day, think of new and more interesting ways to motivate and challenge your partners. Set high goals, encourage competition, and then keep score. Make bets with outrageous payoffs. If things get stale, cross-pollinate; have managers switch jobs with one another to stay challenged. Keep everybody guessing as to what your next trick is going to be. Don't become too predictable.

- Rule 4: *Communicate* everything you possibly can to your partners. The more they know the more they'll understand. The more they understand, the more they'll care. Once they care, there's no stopping them. If you don't trust your Associates to know what's going on, they'll know you don't really consider them partners. Information is power, and the gain you get from empowering your Associates more than offsets the risk of informing your competitors.

- Rule 5: *Appreciate* everything your Associates do for the business. A paycheck and a stock option will buy one kind of loyalty. But all of us like to be told how much somebody appreciates what we do for them. We like to hear it often, and especially when we have done something we're really proud of. Nothing else can quite substitute for a few well-chosen, well-timed, sincere words of praise. They're absolutely free—and worth a fortune.

- Rule 6: *Celebrate* your successes. Find some humor in your failures. Don't take yourself so seriously. Loosen up, and everybody around you will loosen up. Have fun. Show enthusiasm—always. When all else fails, put on a costume and sing a silly song. Then make everybody else sing with you. Don't do a hula on Wall Street. It's been done. Think up your own stunt. All of this is more important, and more fun, than you think, and it really fools the competition. "Why should we take those cornballs at Wal-Mart seriously?"

- Rule 7: *Listen* to everyone in your company. And figure out ways to get them talking. The folks on the front lines—the ones who actually talk to the Customer—are the only ones who really know what's going on out there. You'd better find out what they know. This really is what total quality is all about. To push responsibility down in your organization, and to force good ideas to bubble up within it, you *must* listen to what your Associates are trying to tell you.

- Rule 8: *Exceed* your Customers' expectations. If you do, they'll come back over and over. Give them what they want—and a little more. Let them know you appreciate them. Make good on all your mistakes, and don't make excuses—apologize. Stand behind everything you do. The two most important words I ever wrote were on that first Wal-Mart sign: "Satisfaction Guaranteed." They're still up there, and they have made all the difference.

- Rule 9: *Control* your expenses better than your competition. This is where you can always find the competitive advantage. For twenty-five years running—long before Wal-Mart was known as the nation's largest retailer—we ranked number one in our industry for the lowest ratio of expenses to sales. You can make a lot of different mistakes and still recover if you run an efficient operation. Or you can be brilliant and still go out of business if you're too inefficient.

- Rule 10: *Swim* upstream. Go the other way. Ignore the conventional wisdom. If everybody else is doing it one way, there's a good chance you can find your niche by going in exactly the opposite direction. But be prepared for a lot of folks to wave you down and tell you you're headed the wrong way. I guess in all my years, what I heard more often than anything else was: A town of less than 50,000 population cannot support a discount store for very long. [From *Sam Walton: Made in America*, by Sam Walton. Copyright © 1992 by the Estate of Samuel Moore Walton. Used by permission of Doubleday, a division of Random House.]

Notice that 60 percent of Sam Walton's message was about people management (rules 2 through 7, a picture notably different from the widespread layoffs found in the hospital industry. Should this thinking be dismissed, or could it be that the world's richest man understood something that health care didn't?

And there are plenty of other winning organizations to emulate. They keep turning up in the management journals like *Fortune's* annual list of Most Admired Corporations (Table 6.1). The body of management research published since *In Search of Excellence* (Peters and Waterman, 1984, 1997) has demonstrated that there is a generally common success profile of what such companies do with Customers, Associates, and work systems. Winners, regardless of industry, were more like each other than they were like competitors in their own industry. This pattern of winning served to confirm that we were on the right trail in thinking that the profile might also work in hospitals.

Fortune's 1998 survey showed that none of the best-rated organizations were perfect; none got a "ten" on the eight factors on which they'd been scored. But they were the best in their respective industries—benchmarks nevertheless.

One point of new learning in our work came when we began to understand that health care organizations were going to have to become operationally excellent in their markets. That meant that benchmarking just any excellent organization would not be appropriate. We had to zero in on organizations that were pursuing a similar low-cost orientation. So we began to look more deeply at understanding what benchmark organizations did that might be appropriate in health care. From Table 6.1, those organizations included Coca-Cola, McDonald's, Walt Disney, Home Depot, Southwest Airlines, and Wal-Mart. (Although a ticket to Disney World might not make you think so, Disney is a low-cost producer.)

Table 6.1. Who Do We Want to Be Like?
Fortune's Most Admired Corporations.

- Quality of management • Quality of products/services
- Innovativeness • Ability to attract, develop, keep talented people
- Long-term investment value • Use of corporate assets
- Financial soundness • Community and environmental responsibility

Number	Company	Industry	Points*
1.	General Electric	Electronics/ Electrical Equipment	8.18
2.	Microsoft	Computer Services	8.28
3.	Coca-Cola	Beverages	8.68
4.	Intel	Electronics	8.75
5.	Hewlett-Packard	Computers	7.90
6.	Southwest Airlines	Airline	7.14
7.	Berkshire Hathaway	Insurance	7.78
8.	Disney	Entertainment	7.61
9.	Johnson & Johnson	Pharmaceuticals	7.79
10.	Merck	Pharmaceuticals	7.99

First in industry below Top 10

Number	Company	Industry	Points*
13.	McDonald's	Food Services	7.15
18.	Home Depot	Specialist Retailers	8.07
51.	Wal-Mart	General Mdse	7.23

*Point rankings are not highest to lowest due to complex scoring method.

Being more selective of those organizations pursuing a similar market orientation really sharpened our thinking and made us more rigorous in our recommendations. Though we still look at what winning organizations do that are pursuing a different market orientation, we tend to do so more selectively. For example, Hewlett-Packard is worth examining closely because of their excellent approach to human resources.

Why the New Model Succeeds

The results of trying to install hundreds of these best practices were mostly favorable. The model was tested in approximately 100 hospitals; each successive iteration improved and expanded the number of best practices implemented. Hospitals were given a lengthy action plan with several hundred elements to be inserted, detailed implementation manuals, and fourteen days of intensive management training. They were shown how to do organizational development tasks. In addition, a huge amount of worker input, either in individual assignments known as JDIs (Just Do Its) or in small groups known as DIGs (Do It Groups), resulted in change recommendations within thirty days. The health care organizations that emerged were a blend of best practice ideas, systems, and organizing schemes inserted by consultant intervention plus a more massive flow of internal ideation from managers and Associates.

Figure 6.1 depicts the general framework and conceptualization of the New American Hospital, an organization that is described by seven factors. To function superbly, the organization has to be simultaneously

Uncommonly led

Values driven

Associate powered

Systems controlled

Customer focused

Future creating

Competitively dominant

The work of transformation is to install best practices in each of these areas. Like ingredients in a recipe, the interaction of best practices in each of these segments produces a robust and fully flavored stew. The organizational cook can't leave out some ingredients or use ingredients that are less than the best. The magic of the recipe is how all of these elements combine, often in astounding, always exciting, ways. To illustrate, many Total

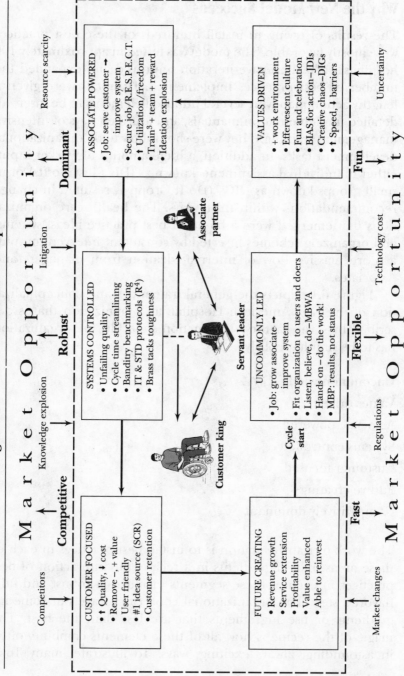

Figure 6.1. The New American Hospital.

Market Opportunity

Competitors — Knowledge explosion — Litigation — Resource scarcity

Competitive — **Robust** — **Dominant**

ASSOCIATE POWERED
- Job: serve customer → improve system
- Secure job/R.E.S.P.E.C.T.
- ↑ Utilization/freedom
- Train^3 + team + reward
- Ideation explosion

VALUES DRIVEN
- + work environment
- Effervescent culture
- Fun and celebration
- BIAS for action—JDIs
- Creative chaos—DIGs
- ↑ Speed, ↓ barriers

SYSTEMS CONTROLLED
- Unfailing quality
- Cycle time streamlining
- Banditry benchmarking
- IT & STD protocols (R^4)
- Brass tacks toughness

UNCOMMONLY LED
- Job: grow associate → improve system
- Fit organization to users and doers
- Listen, believe, do—MBWA
- Hands on—do the work!
- MBP: results, not status

CUSTOMER FOCUSED
- ↑ Quality, ↓ cost
- Remove −, + value
- User friendly
- #1 idea source (SCR)
- Customer retention

FUTURE CREATING
- Revenue growth
- Service extension
- Profitability
- Value enhanced
- Able to reinvest

Associate partner

Servant leader

Customer king

Cycle start

Fast — **Flexible** — **Fun**

Market changes — Regulations — Technology cost — Uncertainty

Market Opportunity

Quality Management (TQM) projects (work in the "Systems Controlled" box of Figure 6.1) failed in hospitals during the 1990s because the supportive precursor elements were not in place. TQM, or other good recipe ingredients, fail because the rest of the stew is missing.

Uncommonly led. Everything begins with leadership, and the performance cycle of the New American Hospital begins there, too. A new leadership model is necessary before the work of organization renewal can go forward. As Dr. Mark Silber said, "Improved organizations, and improved management, come only from improved managers." The primary task for the leader is the growth of her people, which represents the organization's prime competitive advantage (PCA); improvement of the system is a close second. The task of leadership is to change the organization so that it fits what the users need and what the doers require. Rather than rely on policy, the new leader knows that today's solution is to spend a great deal of time interacting with Customers and Associates to listen to their reports, believe them, and then get that work done—taking orders from those on the front line of what the business is all about. In this new leader-as-servant role, leaders work the staff jobs and focus on following management best practices. This means a focus on results, not status. Overall objective: Achieve all the organization's Big Hairy Audacious Goals (BHAGs).

Values driven. The New American Hospital is not market driven but values driven. One of its values is Customer satisfaction, in which we choose to serve the market, not be driven by it. The old repressive culture of yesteryear's hospital is eradicated. In its place is one of celebration for the many achievements—job joy and satisfaction in creative work, where ideas are born and problems killed instead of the other way round.

One way to think of this cultural transformation is that management creates the kind of work environment that makes it possible for people to do their best. Like gardeners preparing the soil, leaders create the conditions that allow the life force of people at work to achieve greatness. As any gardener knows, you can't make plants grow, you can only create the conditions where growth is possible. As the culture again returns to the "family feel" that senior workers often report has been lost, the organization increasingly finds itself able to move quickly to solve problems and reduce barriers. This superior culture becomes ingrained and second nature in twelve to twenty-four months from the start of organizational renewal.

Associate powered. Associates (pejorative language like employees, subordinates, or lower levels is out of touch) are focused on two targets: satisfy their downstream Customers; attack the system by improving it. The strategy is to build a smarter and more able team than competitors' through providing enriched and bigger jobs, lots of training (the first year standard is 40 hours per full-time person), less restrictive supervision, and lots of cross-functional teams. The goal is to create self-directed teams within twenty-four to thirty-six months with a corresponding reduction in the numbers of managers necessary to assist such a powerful workforce. The transaction between Customers and Associates is defined as the primary definition of the business. The power of releasing Associates' intellectual capital fuels competitive advantage. Organizations win only if they are able to release the power of their people's thinking. Overall objective: Achieve the best people BHAG. Finally, we don't "empower" the people, they already have the power. What we need to do is figure out how to stop depowering them and get out of their way.

Systems controlled. This box focuses on all the tasks and projects necessary to streamline work processes. Into this arena is tossed all the reengineering, continuous quality improvement, information technology, cycle time reduction, and standardization of clinical protocols. Overall objective: Achieve the high-quality and low-cost BHAGs. Erring managements most often focus here, failing to put in place the other pieces and failing to understand that there is a sequence of change.

It is here that the organization is creating something which is valued by the market, what they are willing to pay for and prize highly—quality care at affordable prices. Note that this step is impossible to achieve if the previous steps have been short-changed.

Customer focused. Customers are defined in the New American Hospital as the beneficiaries of the work that is done by each jobholder. This downstream orientation determines not only how well present tasks are done, but also defines whether Customer expectations are being met (minimally required) or exceeded (desired). The Customer's primary directives are for higher quality, lower cost, and delightful service. An internal team of "Customer commandos" oversees the installation of all changes necessary to achieve these targets, beginning with a long list of irritations needing removal and an equally long list of value-added ideas that add little or no cost. Overall objective: Achieve the high-satisfaction BHAG.

Future creating. Both profit and revenue growth are the natural outcome of the New American Hospital. Whereas many organizations are preoccupied with financial performance, the new leadership knows that the focus has to be upstream. When the above five factors are attended to, financial vitality results as a natural consequence. This financial health in turn creates future possibilities such as new services, greater community outreach, new technology, and other opportunities. Having earned the right to be at the table, the high-performance organization has the economic vitality and vibrancy to play in the bigger game the future represents.

Competitively dominant. Figure 6.1 shows the difficult and often hostile forces that affect the organization from the outside. Many executives have spent far too much time worrying about these headaches, spending time away from their organizations in various political and lobbying efforts. Very little can be achieved to modify these external forces. The aware leader realizes that the secret is to focus on the variables internal to the organization, most of which are controllable and produce far more powerful forces (indicated by the large outward-pointing arrows). The New American Hospital is competitively dominant. These organizations have typically taken market share and improved measurably over others in their region.

Results of the Model

Results of the New American Hospital model have improved over the years. The more complete the model became and the more thorough the approach to deal with the change problems encountered in dealing with house-wide transformation, the better and more predictable were the outcomes. Currently, a number of the nation's Top 100 Hospitals (published annually by Mercer

Associates with HCIA data) and hospitals rated in the top five percent in Customer satisfaction (on surveys like Press-Ganey) are New American Hospitals.

A case in point is Holy Cross Hospital on Chicago's south side. When it began its effort to transform, the organization was $9 million in the red and its Customer satisfaction score was at the thirteenth percentile according to Press-Ganey. Figure 6.2 shows how Associate ideas affected both Customer satisfaction and financial performance during the first two years of its turnaround effort— a true Cinderella story. The return on investment (ROI) figures reported here show only the financial return from ideas generated, not the bigger picture of other financial improvement stemming from better systems and new service programs.

Press-Ganey reported that they had never seen a hospital move so rapidly from near-bottom to the ninety-seventh percentile (achieved in less than twelve months), nor had they seen a hospital maintain such a consistent high rating month by month after elevating so far (personal communication, 1996, Press-Ganey staff). Named the American Hospital Association's Great Comebacks Award winner in 1994, Mark Clement, the hospital's CEO, reports that in 1994 the organization momentarily took its eye off the Customer, thus causing a slump in ratings, a lesson they have not forgotten.

Note the high number of implemented changes and the tangible return on investment that provided some hard dollars (not all did). And there were lots of other benefits. The chart does not show numerous other positive outcomes, such as lower turnover, higher morale, increased physician satisfaction, and numerous operational and systems improvements. It does demonstrate the direct linkage between a renewed culture and an empowered work force and the direct impacts on business performance.

Although a number of competing management philosophies and practices are currently at work in the industry, those that differ greatly from the New American Hospital are unlikely to succeed. This model is built for speed of response and is highly adaptive at making massive change. It is fast, flexible, and fun; robust and competitively dominant. In some form, it is what most health care organizations will become if they wish to survive in a managed care environment. It works! Focused as it is on benchmark level performance via best practices, it is an organizational

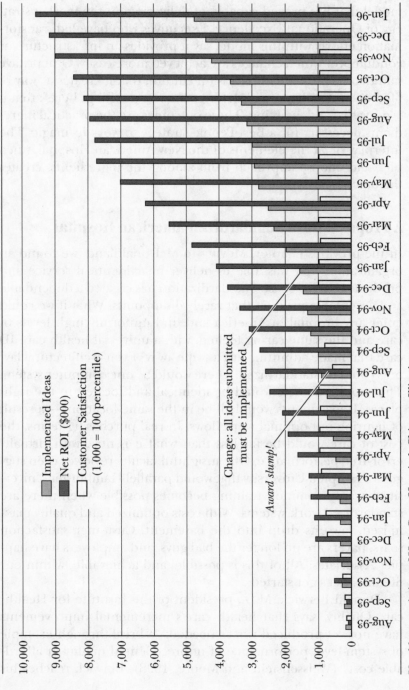

Figure 6.2. Ideation Has an Impact on Holy Cross.

Used by permission of Holy Cross Hospital, Chicago, Illinois.

model that has proved capable of delivering on the market strategy of Operational Excellence. Executives who have led transformation efforts with this model say it provides an infrastructure or conduit over which changes are achieved more easily. Others have said that its ultimate impact is on culture; that it creates a "way of life," an atmosphere, and defines "how we do things here"; that it is pervasive and enabling. These outcomes are the practical ingredients necessary for a Best People strategy to work its magic. The interplay of *all* the elements of the New American Hospital, not a pick and choose approach from among the ingredients, creates the outcomes.

A Proposal for a Standardized American Hospital

In the previous chapter, Moving to McDonaldland, we found an organization that was able to deliver near identical service and products coast to coast. Standardization has created a dependable and acceptable product that rarely disappoints. What if we could enter any hospital in America and find uniformly high levels of care and the same caring feeling, with a universal health care ID card that made admitting just a swipe away? Even architectural layouts could be standardized. There would be one computer system. The supply cabinets would be identical and located in the right places. Departments would all be in the same locations—a result of figuring out optimal work flows. In real purchasing terms, the cost of care would be far less than what it is now, with virtually error-free performance. One insightful faculty reviewer even suggests a Hospital University that would parallel Hamburger University, because common training becomes possible when there are standardized work systems. With costs optimized and quality maximized, lawsuits drop into the basement, Customer satisfaction soars, payers are no longer the bad guys, and employers have happier Associates. All of this is possible, and achievable, within our lifetime. Let's get started.

Donald Berwick, M.D., president of the Institute for Healthcare Quality, says that health care's incremental improvements have not yet produced what's needed: "a breakthrough example of system-level performance of unprecedented quality at affordable cost" (Weissenstein and Moore, 1998). Berwick reaches his conclusion by looking at HEDIS quality measures, which showed little or no progress from 1996 to 1997. Evidence is mounting that squeezing and tweaking the old system as a management approach may have run its course, and that the time has come for some breakthrough thinking and moving to a whole new model, perhaps something along the lines of the New American Hospital.

Although the New American Hospital model has certainly been an improvement over the old, one wonders how much more could be achieved. What if these transformed organizations were used in a national trial as pilot operations in which best practices were installed housewide? The goal of this next step would be to create the best-performing hospitals in America, a full-blown set of examples of complete best thinking at work, with far better performance than any hospital in the world. These would then become the basis for McDonaldland health care. The project would

1. Select one to three hospitals in each of four to six regions to test for size and regional differences. Other selection criteria would include readiness for change and commitment to the concepts of the New American Hospital.
2. Install in every department a full array of best practices. Ideally these would be endorsed by national associations, researchers, and field practitioners; that is, a ratings or approval process would stamp practices as "best of breed."
3. Measure process and business outcomes to show improvement over baselines.
4. Oversee the project. A national steering group would include representatives from all affected parties: providers, government, academia, employers, and professions. This team would be an action-oriented group primarily bent on getting results, not a debating society. Something akin to the Manhattan Project or a NASA moonshot is contemplated.

That we have now reached a point that such a project is feasible is exciting. If we built a set of such organizations, it would make replicating them across the country far easier, and at far lower cost. One-by-one, piece-by-piece organizational renewal is costly and slow. Every hospital right now is reinventing this wheel. It's like making each suit by hand, when a designer-suit right off the rack could be made available nationwide. The next logical step in American health care's evolution is to scale up from the successful but partial examples provided by New American Hospitals. And this should include all health care services and all departments.

The remarkable dream of a total best practices hospital is within our reach, but today's managements cannot wait for its fruition. Making change today in the direction of the New American Hospital with its partial list of best practices is the interim path.

Conclusion

This chapter has summarized the author's experience of helping many hospital managements implement a strategy of best practices applied to major areas of organization performance. This field-tested model validated the notion that changing how an organization functions changes its ability to produce business results. If higher standards are to be reached, there has to be a delivery vehicle that can get us there. The New American Hospital model is such a vehicle.

The New American Hospital is not the apex or ultimate standard, however. Although it is an admirable achievement, a breakthrough benchmark, the New American Hospital is the new minimum standard that managers must create as a platform from which future efforts can be launched. That work will be that of standardization, both creating or implementing the higher standards of best practices and uniformly applying them across systems. In the following chapter we're going to look at how health care's very bright people can be put to work to make this dream possible.

Work-Out Session

1. Identify as long a list as possible of Customer complaints and irritations. These need to be fixed. Typically they have been around for years, a sign of organizational nonresponsiveness. Make a second list of what would add value to the patient's experience. These are not luxury items or new elements of cost. What could be added that would improve the customer's experience?

2. Now do the same for Associates. What irritations need to be removed from the work situation? What improvements need to be added (without adding substantial cost)?

3. Have a third group create a list of problems with work processes, quality, or cost inefficiencies. Where are tools, big and little, needed? Where are waits and delays in the system? Which of these are small issues that could be readily resolved versus major work flow overhauls? (Don't fall prey to fears that everything is a major reengineering problem, requires a tedious use of TQM tools, or can only be resolved by a fifteen-step problem-solving process; 80 percent of problems aren't that complicated.)

4. What is missing in management team performance? What do managers need in the way of new training or increased autonomy and accountability? (Example: if managers need more than one countersignature on requisitions, the system is overly bureaucratic.) What would it take to make the management group a team of champions?

5. What is needed to make a freer and more joyous work environment and culture? List changes that might eradicate interdepartmental segregation, like work rotations, interdepartmental recognition schemes, and organizational achievement celebrations. "All work and no play makes Jack a dull boy." Where would play free up your organization?

6. Experience shows these exercises will usually generate several hundred ideas in an hour. Pick some priorities, and start hacking away.

Chapter Seven

Competing on Knowledge

We are at a turning point in history regarding what determines the success and wealth of organizations. The ways and means by which organizations were judged to be successful in the past have little relevance to what it will take to be successful in the future. Many health care executives are struggling to find new bearings. Old formulas no longer work, and new formulas are hard to come by. This chapter will look at the best new formula around—how to apply intellectual capital to the problems at hand (among the many new texts on the subject, see Edvinsson and Malone, 1997; Klein, 1997; Stewart, 1997).

Brain power. We joke about it because we understand its central importance in our lives. I personally realize that my brain is a wonderful organ: It starts working the moment I get up in the morning and doesn't stop until I get to work. George Carlin says that the average woman would rather have beauty than brains, because the average man can see better than he can think! The joking is fun, but it's no joke when our ideas at work aren't listened to, or our organization rejects our best thinking.

What does it mean to live in the Information Age? What must management do differently in such an age? Alvin Toffler has written that with the explosive emergence of the Information Age the new and dominant form of power is that of *mind. Mind power* eclipses the power of money and economics. Who would have thought twenty years ago that Bill Gates, with a single patent on MS-DOS, was destined to be far wealthier than IBM? Mind power surpasses the power of might and military muscle. To prevail in today's worldwide economy, a nation, an organization, wins only through brain power.

The New Currency of Intellectual Capital

As Drucker has been saying for fifty years, it's important to recognize that we're now managing in an age of discontinuity, in which there is a radical and complete break from the past. We are managing within parameters completely different from those encountered by any generation of leaders before. We are seeing the rise of a new civilization and culture, both nationally and worldwide.

Knowledge is estimated to be doubling every five years; in certain fields, such as electronics, genetics, and other high technologies, knowledge is doubling every 18 months. The organization that can't keep itself "in the know" winds up in a state of ignorance and places itself directly in front of the onrushing information train. The health care organization that wins will be highly skilled at obtaining, disseminating, and rapidly leveraging knowledge for competitive advantage. *Standardizing best practices* is a phrase that translates simply as "the insistent use of the state of the art."

What does that mean for today's health care management, scrambling to keep up with change? How can the concepts of intellectual capital be put to use to disseminate best practices throughout the organization system and to continually elevate the standards of what we do?

The Organization's Most Valuable Asset

Nowhere is the inadequacy of financial measures demonstrated better than in their inability to measure the true worth of the organization—its intellectual assets. The concept has now moved from a sideline discussion on the adequacy of management metrics to center stage in the debate over survival and success.

What Is It?

Fortune's definition is that intellectual assets are the "intangible assets of skill, knowledge, and information" (Stewart, 1994). Clearly, the team that is more skilled and knowledgeable and has greater access to needed information will carry the day. Another definition of intellectual capital is intellectual material that has been formalized, captured, and leveraged to produce a higher-valued asset. The idea that it is possible to add value to the enterprise by getting and leveraging intellectual assets is pure dynamite. We win with our smarts. Consider a hypothetical case of two competing hospitals (see Table 7.1; the statistics are just a snapshot in time). Which organization would you bet on in terms of future performance?

The last three measures of Table 7.1 are gross indicators of the use of intellectual capital. Think of them as drivers or inputs of future organizational performance: They are *leading indicators* of what is going to happen in the organization's future. With higher morale, more training, and the aggressive implementation of Associates' ideas, it is clear that Work Smarter Community is going to overtake its competitor rapidly. The first two measures are outputs of previous performance: They are *following indicators* and come out of past performance. In this case, these financial indicators were subsequently reversed in terms of position. The eventual loser was Sleepy Memorial.

Who Has the Answers for Improvement?

Organizations are profitable and succeed only when they can solve Customers' needs and problems better than their competitors. If organizations existed in a static state, today's answer would still be good tomorrow. When things weren't moving so fast, it used to be possible to hire physicians and other trained people who had a set of answers for problems that would continue to have value for many tomorrows, but that is no longer the case. We must have new answers now for today's new problems. Wrote Drucker: "It is futile

Table 7.1. A Battle of Wits.

Performance Indicator	Sleepy Memorial	Work Smarter Community
Current sales/market share	60M/%	40M/%
Debt	0	9M
Workforce opinion survey	40th%tile	85th%tile
Ideas implemented worker/yr	0.1	4
Training hours/worker/yr	6	40

to restore normality. Why? Because 'normality' is the reality of yesterday. The job is not to impose yesterday's normal on a changed today, but to change the business, its behavior, its attitudes, its expectations—as well as its products, its markets, and its distributive channels—to fit new realities" (Drucker, n.d.).

So, if we need a lot of ideas, and we need them now, where can we turn? The boom in consultant business is directly related to the present emergency, but it results from yesterday's fallacy that somebody, usually outside, has an existing, canned answer. Suppose that answers are a perishable commodity, like freshly baked bread. As a product it's needed, tastes great, but has to be replaced with more fresh baked bread tomorrow. I suppose we could wait for the bread truck to arrive from Boston late next week, or we could go out in the kitchen, gather our people around us, and bake our own bread. Are the people in your organization able to produce your own fresh baked bread?

Organizations must learn how to learn. They must find that they can learn how to solve their own problems—under their own power. Every organization must learn how to exploit its own knowledge and to develop new approaches from its own successes. But these successes often remain overlooked opportunities of which executives are often unaware. In the most troubled health care organizations there are islands of strength—a great program here, a bright person there, brilliant elements of culture buried in the mire. Learning how to find these winning elements, grow them, and spread their influence is what knowledge management is all about.

Turn On the Power of Intellectual Capital

Perhaps the biggest financial mistake of past health care leadership has been the inability to see that most of the answers to their problems were all around them in the people whose opinions were never asked, whose minds found no avenue to assist with solutions. Sony CEO Akio Morita said, "American management's biggest failure is they do not recognize that their prime competitive advantage [PCA] is their people." The nonuse of intellectual capital by executives in the midst of the Information Age probably ought to qualify them for the Dufus prize.

What's an Idea Worth?

Our hospital clients who have been experimenting with human capital management are showing that the return on investment (ROI) of implemented ideas has a value ranging between $1400 to $3000 per idea in the first year of implementation. (We use $2000 as a working average.) This range is calculated by a conservative formula that assumes (erroneously) that there is no value to intangible implemented ideas:

$$\text{AVERAGE IDEA VALUE} = \frac{\text{ROI (hard dollars from tangible ideas only)}}{\text{TOTAL IMPLEMENTED IDEAS (tangible + intangible)}}$$

Many ideas have no tangible financial return (experience has shown these are often the majority of ideas) but they are absolutely valuable and important to the business. Indeed, even blockbuster tangible ideas have sometimes been judged less valuable to the business than some intangible ones. Here are some examples of intangible ideas for which executives reported an *extremely high business value:*

- Two hourly Associates were put on the hospital board. What was the dollar value in terms of staff communication and influence?
- The hospital created a Physician Action Council (PAC). In the first ninety days the group reconfigured medical staff committees so that physicians could spend less time at the hospital, and reduced the time to process credentials of new physicians who were clamoring to get in. What was the worth of creating the PAC?
- A housekeeper suggested placing a rose on the bed so that each admitting patient sees a token of sentiment and hospitality as they enter the room. What is the impact on the organization in financial terms?

It is easy to see both sides of this issue: the problem of measuring the intangibles, and the risk of thinking that there is no true business value in intangibles. Let's be clear: Intangibles are real and valuable, they are just hard to measure. By assuming a conservative dollar value for all ideas, an organization becomes far more ready to listen to the birthing cries of new thinking. When an Associate approaches her manager, saying, "I've got an idea," it's worth at least $2000 to listen.

The second part of the calculation is to determine how many implementable ideas an organization can produce. Our experience has been that a health care organization of 1000 people can easily produce twice their staff count in implemented ideas—that is, two per person—in the first year of effort. If Work Smarter Community Hospital has 1000 people producing 2000 ideas at a value of $2000 each, that equals a value to the organization of $4 million. In the second year, it is possible to increase those numbers in two ways: number of ideas/person, and dollar value per idea through better implementation approaches. A benchmark comparison at Disney is for twelve submitted ideas per person per year. That rate at Work Smarter Community would mean an ROI of $24 million.

The concepts surrounding the use of intellectual capital may seem unusual to some. This is not "funny money," nor is it fanciful or fantastic. Before considering how to make further application, let's get a better handle on defining terms and understanding how the management community is beginning to use these power tools for profit and fun.

Other Estimates of Worth

Intangible measurement is always problematic but worth pursuing. Citibank, the nation's largest bank, estimates that a company's intellectual assets are worth three to four times book value. The London School of Economics states that intellectual assets "exceed many times balance sheet value." The Tuck School of Management at Dartmouth estimates that as much as 75 percent of value added is knowledge-derived. It is clear that an organization's most valuable assets are tied to its use of information and knowledge, most of which is created or acted on by human brain power.

But there is a significant problem in using financial measures designed before the beginning of the twentieth century: They fail to pick up the intangible value of proper management, the economic value added (EVA) by leaders. Without becoming too technical, let's look at the mounting evidence that financial measures are increasingly undervaluing organizational wealth, due to their inability to trace what's been a growing amount of intellectual capital. For example:

• Over the past twenty years there has been a widening divergence between statements of value on corporate balance sheets and investors' assessment of these values (K. Bradley, cited in Stewart, 1997). Calculations for 1992 showed that approximately 40 percent of the market value of the median U.S. public corporation was missing from the balance sheet, rising to over 100 per cent for knowledge-intense corporations.[1]

• Distortions caused by inadequate financial measures are also reflected in American acquisitions. A study of 391 transactions between 1981 and 1993, with a median value of $1.9 billion, showed that the average price of acquisition-to-book value was 4.4; that is, the real values of acquired corporations were about four and a half times larger than the values reported in the balance sheets, and price-to-book values were larger than ten for knowledge-intense companies.

• Substantial evidence shows a declining relationship between accounting data and stock prices and investment returns as the true source of competitive advantage and profit have become more dependent on intellectual capital and intangible assets. About 95 per cent of the differences across firms' ongoing stock price changes are unrelated to earnings.

This weakening relationship between accounting data and capital values suggests that financial reports will have less and less utility to investors (K. Bradley, cited in Stewart, 1997). Stated another way, balance sheets are becoming less informative and even

---

[1] Bradley reports that the median market-to-book ratio for U.S. public corporations over a twenty-year period between 1973 and 1993 increased from 0.82 to 1.1692. He writes: "In knowledge intense industries the often substantial investment in intellectual capital renders accounting matching mechanisms misleading. Unable or unwilling to capitalize and amortize intellectual capital (to match its costs with future benefits) accounting authorities generally mandate the immediate expensing. This depresses current earnings and book values while leaving the subsequent deficits of these investments to be reported without the corresponding costs. In 1992 the median market-to-book value of knowledge intense U.S. corporations was 2.009. This meant that the percentage asset missing from the balance sheet was 100" (cited in Stewart, 1997).

misleading for companies in which intellectual capital tends to be a primary asset.

This clearly means that there are significant "hidden" assets in most American organizations, assets that we currently lack the tools to identify and manage, and this applies to health care organizations as well. As an applied science business, a hospital's very survival has come to depend on its ability to attract and retain the best physicians and many other specialists required by this knowledge-intensive workplace. Less and less can the work of health care be done by people whose minds are not fully employed, degreed or not. The conclusion is inescapable: Intellectual capital management has become a key success factor in the health care industry.

One executive who understands that intellectual capital is the alpha and omega of competitive advantage is Microsoft's Bill Gates. His organization has aggressively recruited and nourished what is widely conceded to be the single most brilliant group of software developers and engineers in the computer industry. Around them he has created an aggressive, flexible, fast, and innovative organization to implement their thinking. The result is domination of the industry. Microsoft's dominance may not sit well with competitors, who are continually being steamrolled by this behemoth, but it is a domination that has been achieved through better use of intellectual capital. Some who are not Microsoft fans would argue that it is not technological or technical superiority but marketing muscle that has accounted for their success. Either way, it is intellectual capital at work.

To illustrate the business value of the new tough-mindedness surrounding the use of brain power at Microsoft, consider where shareholders place its value. With far less in balance sheet assets than IBM, the world's largest computer hardware maker, why is Microsoft, the world's largest software maker, considered to be worth much more than IBM? The answer lies in the value placed on intellectual assets by investors who are betting billions on Microsoft as a category killer, a term used to define dominant players who have no equally powerful rivals (Home Depot and Wal-Mart are other category killers). Figure 7.1 shows the elements of value on a given date of Microsoft's share price. The proportions of value, not the actual share price, are of interest.

Figure 7.1. Why Is Microsoft Worth So Much?

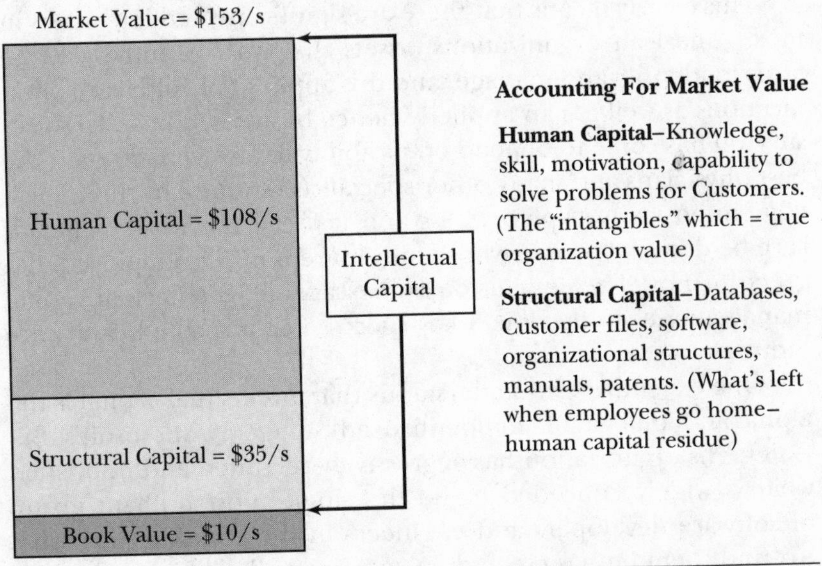

Market Value = $153/s

Human Capital = $108/s

Intellectual Capital

Structural Capital = $35/s

Book Value = $10/s

Accounting For Market Value

Human Capital–Knowledge, skill, motivation, capability to solve problems for Customers. (The "intangibles" which = true organization value)

Structural Capital–Databases, Customer files, software, organizational structures, manuals, patents. (What's left when employees go home– human capital residue)

The message is clear: Management that works to increase book value is working on the short end of the equation. *It's not how many dollars are in the bank, it's how many ideas are in the brains.* The true worth of a business is what it knows and can skillfully deliver. To increase true organizational value, management needs to focus, first, on the growth of human capital and, second, on structural capital, which is a product derived from human capital.

Knowledge Management as New Leadership Task

Since intellectual capital is the raw material from which financial and all other results are made, what must management do? The label that has emerged is *knowledge management*. It is helpful to understand that we do not really manage people, but rather utilize the assets in people: their know-how, skills, and ability to solve problems yet unseen. What are the tasks of the knowledge manager?

1. *Locate intellectual capital.* These assets are scattered, often hidden, and sometimes have two legs, which allow them to walk out the door. They are in to-do lists, old notebooks, on computer

disks. Once found, figure out how to map them, source them. There will be two divisions of this stuff: *human assets,* individuals and teams who can generate ideas; and *organizational structures,* network and dissemination channels. Consider location of intellectual assets to be a best practice.

- Acquire new information and knowledge *external* to the organization. Get it quickly, and as much as possible. Benchmarking, seminars, educational assistance are all approaches to do this.
- Aggressively get all ideas and suggestions for change that *internal* stakeholders have. These would include ideas from Associates, Customers, physicians, and even vendors, who should be considered team members and intellectual partners. Our experience suggests that the greater volume of change ideas will come from these internal sources, rather than from the outside.
- Find out what prevents these ideas from being adopted. Is there a need for in-gathering mechanisms, group processes to polish ideas, or supervisory training so people aren't turned off? If the people have the ideas, how can they be assimilated and used? Think.
- Figure out how to leverage, get more value from, the ideas and knowledge available. A related question is how to spread internally the knowledge you have. Not uncommonly, a solution found for how to handle a problem in one unit fails to spread within the organization, or even within the same unit between shifts.

2. *Measure intellectual capital.* You can't manage what you can't measure. In spite of all the talk of the difficulty of measuring intangibles, it is still doable. Start by counting training hours per person, ideas submitted per person, and ideas implemented per person. Chart the data. Identify units that do the tasks well and benchmark them. Hold contests. Connect these measures to a balanced scorecard approach for the organization. (See the following section on Skandia's approach to measurement and the chapter on balanced scorecards).

3. *Manage human capital.* The task for management is to generate widespread innovation through soliciting ideas, getting staff

to ask questions, encouraging risk taking, and following hunches for improvement. It is possible to grow an organization's human capital by using tactics such as raising hiring standards, intensifying training (business realities, problem solving and continuous improvement (CI) tools, cross-functional teams), redesigning jobs for greater range of experience, and giving rewards and recognition. We have seen workforces come alive as their ideas are listened to and used and they receive widespread recognition and celebration for them. Hospitals that thought they would never get needed training sessions filled by staff, a usual past pattern, found them filled to overflowing after a new job standard was adopted that required a certain number of inservice hours for eligibility for merit increases.

Some of the measures that tell whether you're on target in making progress are quarterly attitude surveys, ideas per person per unit, internal promotion percentage, and turnover rates. Again, experience shows that these statistics move in desirable directions when management encourages the growth of human assets.

4. *Manage structural capital.* Structural capital is seen in the procedures an organization develops over the years, its copyrights, databases, and other forms of intellectual property that have been generated over time. The task for management is to capitalize on these ideas and magnify results from best practices by generalizing them within the organization. Too often ideas are known in one department but not elsewhere, understood on one shift but not on other shifts. Once a better idea or best practice is known, getting the word out and institutionalizing it organization-wide or system-wide becomes the objective.

Customers, the organization's existing relationships with them, knowledge of their current dissatisfactions, and other databases all constitute a part of structural capital. Hospitals that begin to determine Customer wants either by survey or Customer focus groups can move to greater involvement of Customers in problem-solving groups. Tapping Customers' brains is like striking the mother lode. Erosion of market share is not just the loss of finances belonging to the Customer, it is erosion of Customer capital and its value to the business. Zero Customer defections is the goal. Customers either gravitate toward or are repelled by their health care providers. Increasing draw strength and bonding power and adding to relationship loyalties significantly affect Customer capital as part of the overall intellectual capital of the enterprise.

Tools that help turn individual or team know-how into group or system property are e-mail systems, computer networks, searchable internal and external databases, training programs, and continuously updated operating systems with mandatory requirements to use them. Software upgrades are one way to dictate mandatory change without engendering major resistance. Measures that can show progress in this area include number of computers per person, number of implemented ideas per unit, and training hours on new system elements.

5. *Convert human capital to structural capital.* Packaging intellectual capital is another best-practice area. This is where the organization benefits from these assets. Although the costs of setting up the technological and organizational structures are often considerable, they are fast, cheap, and easy to use by others, and it is here that a return on these efforts is generated. The up-front cost pays off down the road. In the early 1990s, Ford Motor Company developed with Texas Instruments an initiative called Managing Knowledge Assets that aimed to make Ford's intellectual capital available through Internet-linking databases around the world. Many other companies are following suit. As one who has had a lifetime supply of hotel experiences, it is still a joy to check into a Four Seasons where I haven't stayed. Within fifteen minutes of hitting the room, I will be contacted by friendly host people to see whether there are updates to my file of preferences (morning paper, wake up time, special menu items), which then become available worldwide within their system.

When packaging intellectual capital, plan to accomplish the following:

- Establish in-house and in-system databases that move past raw information to a how-to-do-it knowledge base. Artificial intelligence and expert systems are a lot more user friendly than having to figure things out from a million unsorted bits of data.
- Intranets and groupware can facilitate information exchange.
- Plan on making substantial investment in programs for skills training and team building.

- Use automatic translation programs of all existing needed processes for the benefit of internal and external human contacts (we live in an increasingly multilingual society).

But remember, as Tom Stewart, editor of *Fortune*, notes: "Intellectual capital is something you can't see, you can't touch, and yet makes you rich" (Stewart, 1997).

Elements of Intellectual Capital

Figure 7.2 shows the components of intellectual capital as conceptualized by Skandia, the international financial services company. This scheme shouldn't be regarded as rigid, for elements might easily be pictured or placed differently. What is most useful about it is that it shows how the various elements relate to each other, and it may help the reader target areas needing more work.

Market value. No longer measured adequately by financial statements, market value comprises the tangible assets or financial capital of the organization and its previously "hidden" value represented by its intellectual capital. Investors have been smart enough historically to figure out the approximate worth of both elements. Invariably, the greater proportion of an organization's worth lies in its intellectual capital, which is missing from the balance sheet.

Figure 7.2. Elements of Intellectual Capital.

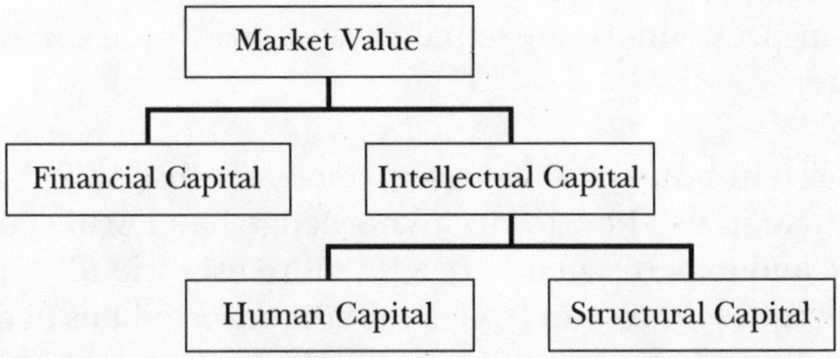

Source: Skandia.

Intellectual capital. The value of the organization's collective human genius and ideation power, and the structural components that represent how human capital has been captured in written documents, procedures, and processes, are summarized under the label *intellectual capital.* Of these two elements, human capital is generally the larger, and by a substantial margin. Management's challenge is to convert as much of the organization's present human capital into the structured form, where it can be preserved, formalized, distributed, and used.

Human capital. Although human capital represents the single greatest asset as a percentage of total business value, it cannot be owned, but can only be rented. It walks out the door every night. This asset can be lost to competitors, depreciated in value through poor motivation and bad leadership, and slowed down or blocked by bureaucratic nonsense (the single best argument against hierarchical forms of management organization). It is also possible for this asset to appreciate in value by hiring smarter and better people, providing skill building, turning people on, speeding up the flow of their thinking, and insisting on better performance by setting high expectations and rewards. In New American Hospital conversions, rapid results have been achieved by going immediately to the people and asking for their ideas for change. An explosion of business value predictably results. When I was a child, I heard the story about the goose that laid golden eggs. I found it very impressive. Years went by and I finally figured out that it's the mind that lays golden eggs. Mind magic. Mind money.

Structural capital. These are the documented and codified approaches that should be taken with customer and operational procedures. This is the distilled wisdom created from human capital, and it represents the platform of current standards and best practices. A common error that organizations make is thinking that instituting best practices via benchmarking is the answer. Although borrowing ideas from the structural capital of other organizations can be beneficial, the benefit is short-lived if human capital in-house is not being developed. The other organizations are continuing to evolve their structural capital, whereas the noninnovative organization is always wearing last year's clothes.

Skandia further divides structural capital into the following components:

- *Customer capital.* Customers aren't just cash boxes, they're partners. Existing relationships and consumers' habitual buying patterns are assets. Customers also are observers of your systems; many are experts in fields which could benefit you. What do your Customers who are teachers, newspaper reporters, and writers think of your communications in-house? Why don't you ask their opinion, or place them on an advisory panel? People aren't just passive patients, they have thoughts that represent value to your business. How can their input be gained?
- *Organizational capital.* Organizational structure, mission, degree of participation, and speed of response are all part of organizational capital. Bureaucratic organizations generally represent a crippled asset in this regard, whereas flatter organizations represent appreciating value.
- *Innovation capital.* Intellectual property, patents, copyrights, and informal solutions that make things work constitute innovation capital. It also includes the intangible assets of morale, teamwork, and spirit.
- *Process capital.* Defined work procedures and processes define how things are done. They were invented or imported by human capital at some point in the past.

Measuring Intellectual Capital

Skandia, the Swedish financial services firm, is the first corporation to create an intellectual capital (IC) report as part of their financial statements (Edvinsson and Malone, 1997). Similar concepts are being used at Citibank, and a host of other organizations are trying to figure out how incorporating such measures might benefit their businesses. An IC report is *not* incorporated into the financial statement, but it can be a lead-in or supplemental report. IC information can be thought of as a predecessor, a predictive function that accounting has never had before. Although the idea of IC measurement may be novel to some, it is being accepted by the Securities and Exchange Commission, a sign of how far down the road of management acceptance the concept has come (Karlgaard, 1997).

Using such an approach before your competitors can yield competitive advantage and provide a far deeper understanding of the organization's operations. Start with two to four measures in each area (financial, Customer, process, renewal and development, human), and build and refine over time. Even the most rudimentary of measures can be of tremendous value. Think about what each measure reveals. You need at least a few indicators to help keep you on top of the boiling cauldron of hot ideas typical of percolating organizations (Malone, 1997).

For instance, under *financial* you might include total assets, total assets per employee, revenues/total assets, revenues and profits resulting from new business operations, revenues per employee, revenues from new Customers compared to total revenues, return on net asset value, return on net assets resulting from new business, investments on information technology, and so forth.

Measures under *Customer* might include market share, number of customers, annual sales per Customer, Customers lost, average duration of Customer relationship, satisfied Customer index, and support expense per Customer.

Process measures might include administrative expense compared to total revenues, PCs and laptops per employee, administrative expense per employee, information technology expense per employee, and corporate performance compared to quality goal.

Renewal and development measures might include competence development expense per employee, training expense per employee, new market development investment, ratio of new product revenue to total revenue, and so forth.

Under *human* measures you might want to list leadership skills index, motivation index, number of employees, employee turnover, average employee years of service with company, percentage of women and minority managers, per capita annual cost of training, communication, and support programs, and on and on.

Figure 7.3 shows the similarity between the market strategy for Operational Excellence enunciated in Chapter Five (high satisfaction, high quality, low cost, best people) and measures of intellectual capital. Organizations in the pursuit of these four primary

Figure 7.3. Managing Intellectual Capital.

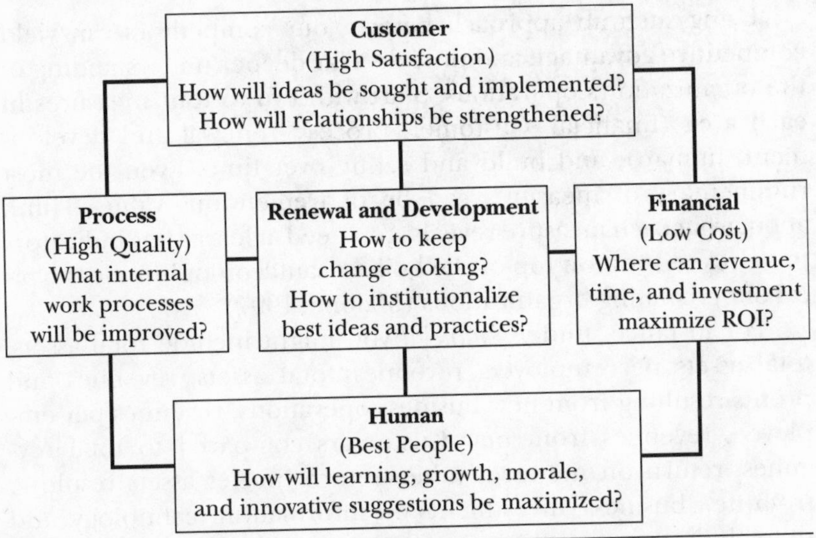

Customer
(High Satisfaction)
How will ideas be sought and implemented?
How will relationships be strengthened?

Process
(High Quality)
What internal
work processes
will be improved?

Renewal and Development
How to keep
change cooking?
How to institutionalize
best ideas and practices?

Financial
(Low Cost)
Where can revenue,
time, and investment
maximize ROI?

Human
(Best People)
How will learning, growth, morale,
and innovative suggestions be maximized?

strategic areas should ask whether intellectual capital is being exploited adequately in each of those areas.

Intellectual capital can be dramatically increased in our health care organizations. Achieving that as a new standard in managing people across American health care will be necessary to survive and thrive.

Computerization and Automation

We come now to the special project needs of computerization, one of the industry's hottest of hot buttons, but we see it in a new light. Computerization and its related cousin, automation, are important for the new millennium because they are tools for better utilization of intellectual capital. Specifically, we should categorize computerization as process capital in the Skandia scheme, a subset of organizational and structural capital. It is simply infrastructure that provides real time data for minds at work.

The degree of penetration of computerization remains disappointingly low in health care when compared to other industries, even though it is one of the most important tools to aid in furthering quality and lowering cost. For perspective, if one picks 1960 as an arbitrary starting line, when "big iron" mainframes had arrived in force in many industries, computerization is a forty-year-old technology—one that is still woefully underutilized or missing in many hospital applications. Decisions not to implement in past years, in some cases by executives who were computer illiterate, now create a steeper learning curve for management to deal with, along with a substantially greater capital investment.

Lack of computerization and the related damage to operations can be seen in many hospitals where department managers report either no computer at all to use, one that is out of date, or inadequate or old software. Another common problem is a lack of interdepartmental connectivity, with only certain departments linked due to incompatibility problems in either hardware or software.

The goal is seamless connectivity, with all system units able to access data via best tools and software applications, information adequately protected, and sufficient flexibility by end users. Standardization of equipment, protocols, and software applications is clearly a winning strategy to achieving these ends. This will be a huge task. A look at how things are progressing does not reveal an entirely happy picture.

Most hospital-centered networks have focused their computerization efforts on departments that cover inpatients. This makes some sense in that inpatients generally have more acute needs, and information system technology was historically present in these departments, thus providing a base on which to build. However, inpatients represent only 30 percent of business volume, and often there is virtually no computerization to monitor the 70 percent of business volume in outpatient clinics and physician offices (Morrissey, 1998a).

With the entry of the Internet as a major new communication highway in 1996, hospitals often lacked the technology to take advantage of it—yet its capability to act as a transfer mechanism between variant hardware and software is unparalleled. Internet software and technologies offer a relatively simple solution to exchanging useful information between computer systems that are otherwise incompatible. Yet one report indicated that only half of provider and payer organizations had designated the Internet as a top priority for the following three years, a third indicated no interest in increasing use of the Internet, and 60 percent have not even articulated a strategy to use the Internet at all. Ninety-two percent of respondents reported confidentiality and security concerns as the reason for not using the Internet—a total disconnect from reality, for security is a nonissue technologically (Morrissey, 1997a).

Given all these problems, why should health care aggressively pursue automation, computerization, and information systems? The answers lie in a potential savings of millions of dollars and huge gains in quality of care. Industry at large went through the inevitable birth pangs of computerization a number of years ago. Questions were raised then about where the payoff was: The perception was that hundreds of billions of dollars were being invested in computer technology without getting significant output gains. This so-called "productivity paradox" was explained by research done at the Massachusetts Institute of Technology Sloan School of Management and reported in *Fortune*—there wasn't one. The Fortune 500 companies they investigated earned "an eye-popping 67 percent return after depreciation on their investments in information technology" ("The Big Payoff from Computers," 1994). In a related study, the U.S. Commerce Department concluded that most of the productivity gains experienced nationally from 1985 to 1994 were due to the huge investment that American businesses poured into computers and other labor-saving technology (Memmott, 1995). This isn't an argument that all computer budgets should be approved, only that the significant gains that will be realized in health care will tend to emerge through time; many will not be visible until what can be a massive infrastructure is built. When did we gain the massive advantages of the nation's interstate system? After we had invested a half trillion dollars.

Here are some examples of how these gains have and will be realized:

- Bedside computers in the ICU at Lutheran Hospital-LaCrosse (Wisconsin) reduced paperwork by 22 percent. This resulted in nurses spending twice as much time assisting patients with daily living activities such as bathing. Staffing levels could be reduced the equivalent of one RN per shift, a net savings of $40,000. An additional benefit for quality "showed a 50 percent increase in information recorded per patient and an improvement in its accuracy" ("Bedside ICU Computers Aid Direct Care," 1991).

- According to research done at Indiana University, computer-using doctors significantly reduce medical costs when ordering drugs and tests electronically rather than by other means. Costs were 13 percent lower per hospital admission. The computer not only provided instantaneous information flow, which speeded results, but also showed physicians side-by-side costs of tests being ordered. The researchers' conclusion on this 5000 patient study was that potential savings could amount to tens of billions of dollars (Winslow, 1993).

The conclusion: Computerize everywhere and quickly for improvements in both quality and cost. Kaiser Permanente, the nation's largest HMO, may be a health care industry benchmark. Their efforts at system-wide computerization were described by *Fortune* as helping to "spark medicine's overdue digital revolution." Their investment is expected to run as high as $1.5 billion to put on line all data affecting their nine million covered lives ($166/person). The system will electronically link its 10,000 doctors and other care providers, and will keep records in a standard digital format. Here are examples of what the system will do in meaningful terms. The computer will

- Remind doctors to prescribe aspirin for cardiac patients to ward off heart attacks and avoid costly emergencies.
- Ask doctors to rank the risk of leg amputation faced by diabetic patients and automatically refer them to podiatry for instruction about foot care. One Kaiser operation saw a 20 percent reduction in amputations based on this feature.
- Remind doctors automatically when patients are due for mammograms.
- Make ordering of all lab tests, searches of medical textbooks, patient referrals, and medication possible online.

- Make formerly bulky patient records available in concise print-outs, and automatically update each new record (Schonfeld, 1998).

Risks of Computer Deployment

Smaller HMOs and health systems may not find it as easy to keep up with the new information management standards being set at the Veterans Administration (VA) Hospitals and Kaiser. Their pockets may not be as deep, and their control over various pieces of the system may not be as extensive.

There are also the risks of project management. According to a report, "Redesigning Health Care for the Millennium," sponsored jointly by VHA and Deloitte & Touche (cited in Pallarito, 1997), a number of managed care plans and health providers have experienced huge problems as a result of computerization efforts. "Many integrated delivery systems have made major investments in facilities and personnel, which give them fixed costs and make them susceptible to disappointing operating performance" (Pallarito, 1997). Deploying vast computer systems is risky. Oxford Health Plans suffered a financial meltdown after a new billing system ran amuck (Schonfeld, 1998). A similar problem occurred with PacifiCare Health Systems when a computer system change-over problem caused a claims backlog (Kertesz, 1997). In the Columbia restructuring from 1997 to 1998, dozens of hospitals marked for spinoff found themselves deeply dependent on the company's electronic infrastructure (Morrissey, 1997b).

Clearly, the argument that a high-performing, standardized information management system should be created in each location is causing a great deal of unnecessary work and great cost. A national project in this area, with output provided to all health providers, would have been more efficient—another opportunity, lost by government and industry leadership.

In arriving at rational plans for computerization, a number of issues will have to be resolved:

- *Tie dollars to clinical results.* The ideal design for a health care information system should integrate clinical as well as administrative and financial applications. Hospitals presently are primarily in the latter two categories. The clinical piece is centered around patients and consists of nursing and nonnursing departmental systems, such as radiology and pharmacy. The key issue is how to integrate digital data so that it can be retrieved anywhere, anytime. This process has begun at Intermountain Health Care, where estimates are that integration will reduce costs by 10 percent for a savings of $100 to $150 million over five years. Substantial benefits are achieved when the information system can produce specific, service-related information. For example, *Modern Healthcare International* reported that 10 percent of mothers discharged after 24 hours had to be readmitted and ended up costing more than if they had stayed an extra day ("IHF Congress Highlights," 1997).

• *Focus on patient data.* The VA's system of 173 hospitals, 800 total facilities, began rolling out a new computerized patient records system in 1997. Expected savings in time and cost are staggering. What is more important, the knowledge for patient care is tremendous. The VA believes its new system may represent the current national standard and may be a useful benchmark. VA doctors who have tried the system report substantial time efficiencies, and the VA sees it as a major tool in its goal to reduce patient treatment costs by 30 percent (Gardner, 1997).

• *Create information clearinghouses to identify best practices.* Twenty-three children's hospitals participate in an information sharing cooperative via the Internet. Known as the Benchmarking Effort for Networking Children's Hospitals (BENCH), the project allows for the trading of information on more than 150 performance indicators. Best performances can then be identified and a closer look given to how they were achieved. An example of how the system works: One hospital had seventy-one lab tests per adjusted discharge; via BENCH information test volume was reduced by half (Morrissey, 1997c).

Information management professionals are doing a good job at information sharing in the industry, thus making efforts easier and collaboration possible. The Health Information and Management Systems Society conducts annual surveys to find out which elements of the overall problem are being attacked and forecasts priorities for the future (Health Information and Management Systems Society, 1998). In reading these reports, one is left with a sense of the many elements that are being pursued. There is an explosion of work in progress to cover many unsolved problems. For instance,

- Only 2 percent of survey respondents say their organizations have a fully operational computer-based patient records (CPR) system in place, and only an additional 34 percent have developed an implementation plan for such a system or have begun to install hardware and software for it. It looks as though CPR is still a distant goal.
- Budgeting both capital and operations technology remains a high concern, along with administrative resistance. Does this suggest a lack of buy-in on the part of administration? Interestingly, in a different survey conducted by *Modern Healthcare,* CEOs are now authorizing 2 percent or less on information systems, without much enthusiasm or confidence in results— a number thought too low by experts, so the technology stagnation continues (Morrissey, 1998b). Perhaps investment in information technology should be thought of as a replacement for the money that used to be budgeted for facilities building and repair. In the new millennium we will need facilities less than we need managed information.
- Security concerns, use of intranets and the Internet remain issues, but solutions remain relatively unsophisticated. Many hospitals haven't even got e-mail up and running. There is a long way to go.

Here Come the Robots!

Automation, whereby computers drive robots, is rapidly moving from something on the sci-fi horizon to a present reality. One of the most notable examples is a pharmacy automation system developed by McKesson Corp. The machinery, installed in approximately 100 hospitals by 1999, tracks inventory, physically fills patient orders on demand, and handles inventory problems. No more does the problem of right label on wrong container, or right pill in wrong bottle, have to worry pharmacy professionals. McKesson claims the robot system is error-free in dispensing 50 million drug doses (Hensley, 1998a).

As information systems and computerization upgrading continue, there will be more capability for other spinoff tasks. Robots have been successfully used by the Navy to deliver in-house supplies. Vanderbilt has used them to feed patients. Tasks that are repetitive, follow consistent travel routes, or are associated with lower skill levels are all tasks that may yield to some form of automation.

But robots will be involved in higher order tasks as well. Star Wars seems to have come to medicine with R2 Technology's ImageChecker, a computerized system that analyzes mammograms and highlights suspected clusters or lumps. It is believed that the system — a support to radiologists, not a replacement for them — could spot 13,000 cancers that would otherwise be missed for every 100,000 currently found during screening. The machine picks up about 83 percent of cancers found by radiologists, and 85 percent of those that people missed on the first screening (Hensley, 1998b). There is little doubt that this robot tool will work its way into use, particularly as unit cost drops.

The potential gain in use of intellectual capital is immense because brain power is freed up to do other tasks. Computerization and automation are only tools to assist health care workers. From a management perspective, the primary need remains how to better utilize staff's intellectual capital.

Conclusion

Health workers will be seen less as a pair of hands and more as a working intellect in the twenty-first century. The concepts of intellectual capital have already demonstrated that most of our health care organizations' worth lies in the minds of its people, a resource too long underutilized. Managements that can create true learning organizations — sending people out to learn and apply — will win. People make the difference, but they make that difference because they create the best thinking.

In the often problem-plagued work climate of the old organization, morale problems and other barriers may prevent the release of best thinking. The next chapter will look at what is necessary to create the kind of place where people can make their full, and best, contribution.

Work-Out Session

1. Do the math. How many people are on your organization's payroll? Assume you can implement two ideas per person and that each idea is worth an average of $2000. Is the resulting number big enough to get management's attention? Assume further that an upper limit based on other industry benchmarks is around 12 per person per year. Somewhere in that range is the annual loss to your business's bottom line.

2. At a management meeting, identify all the barriers to a widescale ideation and implementation approach. What would it take to overcome these very real obstacles?

3. Create a list of all the support elements that would be necessary to make improvement of intellectual capital work. Example: New American Hospitals find that their financial accounts undergo dramatic shifts. Training costs to support Associate empowerment, and development costs to implement new ideas, increase dramatically. Concurrently, consultant fees, legal liability costs, and operating inefficiencies drop substantially as new ideas benefit the system. What would it take to make release of ideation work in your organization?

4. Beyond the grandiose goal of the perfect information system, what practical here-and-now improvements in the information system would help get things done? What affordable hardware and software tools are needed by department? What training in how to use the tools is required?

5. Is working on the intellectual capital concept a *good idea* for your shop? Is this a good idea *now*?

6. What measures are needed to make this issue come alive and to manage it?

Chapter Eight

First Feed the Troops

Any military officer knows that in war the troops get fed first. You can't win without the army, and they're an officer's first accountability. Something has gone terribly wrong in how people are managed in health care, something that flies in the face of the realization that these same people represent the organization's future survival and prosperity. It is essential to understand this failure to lead health care workers well if we are to turn things around and begin to utilize their magnificent capabilities.

Research on worker motivation reveals that people who enter health professions have higher than average scores on benevolence and are motivated by a desire to do good as well as a desire to do well: They want to make a contribution. Surely there are few workplaces that offer more meaningful work, a prime driver of motivation, than does health care. Why then do we see declining morale scores and increased unionization and turnover in this industry? Why is it that only one-third of all trained RNs are still working in their profession?

As a young student I worked in one of those factory jobs one gets to pay the bills while going to school. My coworkers and I had a boss who had learned the difference between theory X and theory Y, and settled on a leadership style that could only be described as theory X^2! On his daily rounds he would "motivate" us by saying, "I'm the boss . . . you're nothin'. I'm the boss . . . you're nothin'." And under our breath we'd say, "Big deal. Boss over nothin'." Such are some people's careers.

Let there be no doubt: World-class health care comes only from world-class work environments, and poor treatment of people will never result in higher standards of service. The Operational

Excellence strategy requires a best-people orientation. There is no winning without them.

When People Were Forgotten

Any serious examination of articles written in the health care press, topics found in health care seminars, or objectives listed in countless health system strategic plans would find heavy doses of system integration, financial issues, reengineering, and customer satisfaction, but precious little content concerning the one element on which all the others depend—people. We will make the case that good people management produces better business outcomes and demonstrate that the Operational Excellence goals of high satisfaction, high quality, and low cost are all driven by best people. We'll first look at what hasn't worked in people managing, and then look at the path of success found by effective leaders. Their results provide ample evidence of the need for the contrarian approach of putting people first and raising standards second.

Layoffs as a Failed Business Strategy

The copycat decision by many old-style hospital administrators and bean counters to reduce costs via layoffs ripped the unwritten contract of trust that long existed between health care employers and their staffs. This ignorance has created a disaster, and its poisons will stay in the soil of the workplace for years. The resultant job insecurity and paranoia has been a predictable result. In one organization conference, a CFO whose prior work experience must have included a stint in a stalag, referred to staff as "disposable units of cost," one of the more stomach-turning labels ever applied to human beings. Research shows that health care workers were seldom asked by management for ideas for cost reduction, even when they were facing the need for dramatic financial cuts—a strategic business error we will revisit later on. More enlightened leaders tried better routes of attrition or early retirement to reduce payrolls because of lowered census.

Still, we have inherited the whirlwind, a human resources tragedy of the highest order that will haunt industry leaders for years in terms of lessened cooperation, unionization, and the loss of many of today's bright young people who will not seek careers with us. What passed as conventional wisdom in the health care industry was nothing more than poverty of thought among a group of people who didn't know how to manage. The greater management community rejects this destruction of intellectual capital. Listen to Jack Stack, CEO of Springfield Remanufacturing Corporation and author of *The Great Game of Business* (Stack, 1996):

> I have no patience with CEOs who make excuses for layoffs, who say they're cutting jobs only to make the company more competitive in the future, to protect the interests of shareholders, to avoid bigger layoffs down the road, or whatever. The implication is that, by downsizing, the CEOs are just doing their job and earning their salaries.

> Bullshit.

> Layoffs are a sign of management failure. You lay people off when you've screwed up, when you've guessed wrong about the market, when you haven't anticipated some critical development or created adequate contingency plans. Reality comes along, smacks you in the head, and forces you to cut costs. Most managers will look for any other cost they can cut before taking away people's jobs. When downsizing is the only choice, it's a sign of how badly management has failed, and the people who get hurt are invariably those who had nothing to do with creating the problems in the first place.

> Let me add that I realize there are times when a company has no choice but to downsize, regardless of who's to blame or what the consequences may be. . . . But that doesn't mean we as business people have to buy into the crazy notion that layoffs are all right. . . . There's something seriously out of whack about that whole way of thinking. [Reprinted with permission of *Inc.* magazine, Goldhirsch Group, Inc., 38 Commercial Wharf, Boston, MA 02110. "Mad About Layoffs" (excerpt), J. Stack, May 1996. Reproduced by permission of the publisher via Copyright Clearance Center, Inc.]

Turnover and morale have long been valid indicators of things gone wrong in the work environment. A comparison of hospital scores to the much more positive worker ratings in related industries such as high-tech (Hewlett-Packard) and hospitality (Four Seasons) reveals that something is clearly wrong. There, innovative and empowered jobs, profit sharing, reduced status differentials, and other approaches have people charged up. Any business that is staffed with the disheartened, the under-educated, warm bodies putting in their time, is not likely to produce competitive advantage or make progress. One of the hallmarks of nonexcellence is a dispirited people, a sad state of affairs that reveals less about the people and more about a management philosophy in serious disrepair.

Staff cuts occurred in 34 percent of hospitals in 1995 and 36 percent in 1996; 28 percent planned to reduce in 1997. Projections are for fewer cuts in the immediate near term, since most of the "fat" has been squeezed out. But how have these cuts affected the rest of the workforce? Although 67 percent of hospitals reported that morale was the major human resource concern in 1994, 86 percent reported it as the prime issue in 1996, and 81 percent as the prime issue in 1997. Concerns being voiced by staff are uncertainty about health care reform, changes in job duties, layoffs, and lack of effective communication (Moore, 1996). Clearly, whatever financial advantages that came from reducing the workforce are diminished by the demoralization this approach has caused. Notwithstanding that layoffs are necessary in some circumstances, it has been instructive to see that a number of health care leaders have held the line. Rather than laying Associates off, they have chosen to involve them in the problem of how to cut costs, and responded by growing out of the problem by creating new business volume with a better product.

Layoffs in the 1980s and 1990s were widely implemented by those governed by the tyranny of numbers. But what are the facts regarding the effectiveness of such an approach? *Money* magazine reported the findings of financial analysts that on average a 10 percent workforce reduction yielded only a 1.5 percent reduction in operating costs, since overtime, separation payments, loss of customers, and other impacts of the layoff rippled through the company. The hoped-for benefits were ephemeral. The average stock performance of downsized companies increased only 4.7 percent after three years, whereas competitors that didn't reduce staff (but did pursue other cost controls) saw their stock increase an average of 34.3 percent. Which stock would you buy? Managements that did layoff workers but then increased training budgets heavily to support the remaining workforce were twice as likely to report improved profits (79 percent) and productivity (70 percent) as those that didn't make this follow-on investment in people. A major conclusion was that layoffs, which make it look like management is taking strong and decisive action, misleadingly inflate current reported profits and tend to divert attention away from the underlying problems eating at the firm's future ("Invest in Companies that Invest in Workers," 1996).

One remarkable study reported that executives often shrink the company because they don't know what else to do. Not understanding how the business should really be run, they panic and execute what is most often recommended by number crunchers—a staff cut. In subsequent periods, the business tends to do no better because root problems are still not fixed, thus leaving the decision maker no other thought but to repeat the cycle of pain, like a drug addict going back for more. (Apply this logic to your family: When times are tough, tell the two oldest kids to get out.) Eventually, when the business has been run into the ground, a new executive is hired to salvage what's left. Said one hospital CEO who succeeded in avoiding a layoff: "Perhaps hospitals would benefit from having a new layoff policy—persons who recommend a layoff will be!"

Granted that many health care organizations needed to right-size given the huge shifts in market conditions, it is important that we reach unequivocally the conclusion that this problem was badly handled. As one of the wisest people I ever knew said, "BS other people if you have to, but never BS yourself." In the eyes of the labor market, this was not just a financial or personnel question, it was a values violation.

Consider what might have happened in hospital organizations had they instituted a practice of cross training so that people could have been used more flexibly and had found ways of opening up the organization to workers' ideas. Several studies reported in *Fortune* of organizations that experienced severe cost management problems but turned to workers for solutions, rather than turning on them, showed that cost improvements were dramatic (see Table 8.1; "What Flexible Workers Can Do," 1989):

Table 8.1. Cost Impacts of Cross Training.

Company	Methodology	Results
Chrysler	Flexible rules, job movement Cross-utilize tradesmen	30% cost reduction
Motorola	Inspection tied to production Salaries tied to skills learned	Defect rate fell 77% Won Baldrige Award
National Steel	Consolidated 78 jobs into 16 Broader responsibilities	22% Productivity increase 33% Customer rejections reduced
Lechmere	Salaries tied to skills learned	Higher Productivity 60% Full-time vs. 30% industry avg

A Body Is Not a Nurse

As many organizations cut back on their payroll, the long-standing problem of unlicensed nursing assistants and other health personnel became more acute. The desire for all-RN nursing staffs, an earlier nursing movement, had proved economically impossible in most locations. Now downsizing often reduced the ratio of professional nurses (registered nurses and licensed practical nurses/vocational nurses [RN and LPN/LVN]) to the unlicensed. Further risks were taken as patient care duties were expanded for the unlicensed, and RNs had to spend more time in supervision rather than in direct patient care. At the heart of the issue is a standards question: How do we assure that unlicensed workers are qualified for the tasks they perform and that they have adequate supervision?

According to one news report, the Institute of Medicine, a health policy group, studied the question of whether the mix of different nursing personnel was affecting quality of care. They were unable to conclude that a problem existed because of the lack of empirical data (Anderson, 1996). Anecdotal data, however, seems continuously to raise the issue with one dramatic event after another reported in the press of adverse patient impacts ranging from patient drops to rape. The Institute of Medicine expressed shock at the "lack of systematic and ongoing monitoring and evaluation of the effects of organizational redesign and reconfiguration of staffing on patient outcomes" (Anderson, 1996).

The layoff question has also revealed other problems. Lawsuits have been initiated by Medicare against some providers for fraud over staffing levels. Since the agency is paying for services (ostensibly defined as so many caregiver hours per case), when those hours are not delivered by short-handed staffs a condition of fraud exists; that is, payment is received for service not rendered. On a related issue, one study found that increasing RN time a half-hour per day resulted in decreases in pneumonia (−4.2 percent), urinary tract infections (−4.5 percent), and thrombosis (−2.6 percent) (D. Moore, 1998b). Though the study was controversial, the whole question of where to make cuts and by how much is at the core of determining proper staffing levels. Clearly the answer is not to just throw more hours at the problem, for that ignores cost, but layoffs where correct staffing is undetermined carries with it a dangerous risk, a case that might be difficult to defend in court.

None of this even touches the even more difficult problem of temporary staff-reliefing, whereby outside agencies send in staff the hospital doesn't know, didn't select, and often doesn't orient. Walt Bogdanich's (1991) critical book, *The Great White Lie: How America's Hospitals Betray Our Trust and Endanger Our Lives,* documents what he calls "cutting corners" and "plugging holes" in this unregulated manpower arena. His view is that there are "absent watchdogs," that no one deals with the issue—not supervision, not regulators. Even the kindest observer of the industry would conclude that in a work setting without standards of training, measurement of learning, and common agreement as to what tasks unlicensed staff should be allowed to perform, we probably won't achieve the kind of patient care that patients need and want.

Labor Speaks Up

No one had to be a psychic to predict that rounds of downsizing and hospital closures and mergers would result both in future labor shortages as young people heard of layoffs and in a resurgence of unionizing activity. When people aren't protected by management, they will seek that protection in other ways. Beyond the political force that unions represent, they also represent a way in which health care workers can voice legitimate concerns over patient care standards. It's hard to be an individual whistle blower; it's a lot easier to be heard when a union raises a collective voice. Although unions can be self-serving (aren't they supposed to be?), listen to what the message of unionized Associates is these days:

• According to a poll of 1,232 workers in various health occupations conducted by the Service Employees International Union (SEIU) and reported in *Modern Healthcare,* over half think quality of care is declining, primarily due to understaffing ("Quality of Care Declining," 1998). Fact: 60 percent of facilities did cut staffing during 1995 and 1996 ("Sixty Percent of Facilities Cut Staffing —Study," 1997).

• Andrew Stern, president of SEIU, the nation's largest health care union, with more than a million members, took the position that the JCAHO should forfeit its "deemed" status under Medicare and Medicaid. The SEIU recommended that the JCAHO should solicit worker advice during accreditation surveys, and that records be kept of actions workers were asked to take to prepare for a survey (Moore, 1997a).

• In Chicago, the SEIU Local 73 pledged to document any unsafe staffing situation at any Chicago health care facility. Part of the controversial program was a "quality care report form" that allowed employees to indicate that they had not been trained on equipment or oriented to an area or procedure, or that they felt the assignment was not consistent with staffing guidelines provided by the Illinois Department of Professional Regulation (Moore, 1997b). Where's management?

• The SEIU showed its dramatic clout when a hospital, previously JCAHO-accredited with commendation, had its rating reduced after four Type I violations occurred. In that case, the SEIU became convinced that surveyors were not seeing real conditions, and that workers' input would be necessary to get a true picture. At least part of the problem stems from the faulty assumption that hospitals maintain good conditions between surveys. Only when the JCAHO came in on an unannounced visit were some of the deficiencies caught (Moore, 1997c). Key point: No matter how much the union was maligned by management, the workers were vindicated—their standards of conduct were higher than management's.

Regardless of one's opinions regarding unions, there are valid lessons to be learned from them that might otherwise remain unheard except through their powerful agents. Regardless, the effective leader knows that to lead the parade you have to get out in front of the band. Clearly there is a need to bring caregivers into the center of both standard setting and monitoring. Their involvement can tremendously help management drive performance upward.

Some of my earliest research was on the question of how unionization could be prevented (Sherman, 1969). The picture then still applies today. Unionization primarily results from a failure of management. It is management's responsibility to represent workers' interests. That a third party must be sought to advocate workers indicates significant social structure breakdown at work.

In those early career years, I was assigned to do attitude opinion surveying. I was struck with the difference in feeling between the cold and lifeless tabulated data that resulted from standard questionnaires and the comments made in small groups where that data came to life through energetic discussion. In group after group I witnessed a full range of emotions: frustrations with supervisors, complaints about training or job assignments, the inevitable gripes about salary (is anybody paid enough?), and a sense of people caught in an organizational web over which they felt largely powerless. Of greater alarm were their reports of problems in work systems that threatened patients' lives, of ideas neglected, of initiatives blunted. It was clear there were two primary problems: how to create a more positive place in which people could feel a sense of achievement and motivation, and how to take their thinking and creative energy and put it to work to benefit the organization's need for improvement. And where was management in all this? Why was I being paid to do management's listening?

Time Warping in the Land of Questionable Standards

As I write this book I am struck with how little has changed in terms of how people are utilized in health care. In 1965 I was a college student in Utah, about to enter the world of work in one of the nation's hospitals for the first time. I was hired based on my application form and positive references. There was no interview.

I had no previous experience working in hospitals or in any job requiring similar skills.

I was assigned to the operating room (OR) where I was to work as a surgical orderly doing tasks such as patient transport, inventory stocking, scrubbing down beds, taking vital signs. I received no formal orientation or training. "Follow Harry around. He'll show you what to do." Harry did show me what to do. He drank on the job, showed me how to do creative accounting on time slips, and the best places to hide out when people needed assistance. It didn't take long to conclude that I needed a different mentor.

I ran frequent trips to the blood bank. I wondered why it was located at the other end of the building from where its product was often needed, immediately. These trips required me to put on an external green robe to cover my OR clothes, but I noted I was moving from unsterile outside departments into the OR area, thus increasing risk of infection. Now, more than thirty years later, these errors continue to be made in many hospitals. Clearly, work systems need to be rethought, and the idea of letting untrained and largely unskilled workers loose in the OR is ludicrous.

Fast forward ten years: In 1975 I was director of human resources for Upjohn Healthcare Services, the first national home care and hospital staff relief enterprise. Ed Wilsmann, a brilliant, multimillionaire entrepreneur, called me into his office and gave me the assignment to set up a standard training program for nurse aides that could be administered nationally in our 230 offices. The problem was twofold:

- There was no nationally recognized job description or training curriculum of what aides were supposed to do. A lot of controversy existed between professional groups as to which tasks could safely be done.
- There was a huge problem of task overlap between jobs in nursing, which indicated problems of job design. Our studies showed nurse aides doing about 58 percent of the tasks done by RNs, while licensed practical nurses did 78 percent. These large percentages were typically being done by aides either with no training or in short training programs of two to six weeks (Sherman, 1974).

Today, we're still handicapped by the lack of national standards as to training content and course length, and we still lack standard measurement to assure learning. We limp along without viable certification, licensure, and accreditation approaches, yet unlicensed workers typically represent half of all nursing personnel in hospitals and more than half in nursing homes. Although Congress passed a 1987 law to establish training standards for nursing homes, they neglected hospitals. Now, a quarter century later, many of these problems persist. Think of it: A large percentage of the hours and interactions with health care's Customers are with people with little standardized training or defined performance expectations.

The Pew Health Professions Commission issued a report calling for all health care professions to be held to national standards for education and credentialing as well as regulation. It calls for the creation of national scope-of-practice guidelines as well as competency standards (D. Moore, 1998a). Clearly we are moving toward the removal of the underqualified and unqualified caregiver. Efforts continue to move in that direction for physicians. A federal credentialing program is being developed that will allow all federal agencies to share verified data on physicians' education, certification, and work experience via the Internet. This will bring together a hodge-podge of programs currently existing in the military, VA, NIH, Indian Health Service, and other sites. The government is working with various software companies to encourage a standardized credentialing report that could be used nationally (Jaklevic, 1998). These are harbingers of what will become a standard national registration of all health workers, a tool that will help protect patients and employers from the incompetent.

One of the curatives to remedy the problem of untrained and unskilled workers in health care may be the National Health Care Skill Standards Project, a collaborative endeavor among health services, labor, and educators. The basic goal is to define the specific training content needed for each health care task. A job can be thought of as a long list of specific tasks. Each task can be defined, the procedure standardized on best practice and best knowledge, training guides prepared, and measures of competency created. Currently, sixty occupations have been included.

National skill standards provide common language and concepts around a number of issues of manpower development and provide benefits to a range of stakeholders:

- Employers recruit, screen, and place potential employees more efficiently
- Workers are better prepared for jobs and career development, thereby fulfilling employer expectations and increasing their chances for mobility and advancement
- Labor organizations maximize the employment security of their members through enhancing education, creating portable skills, and providing opportunities for career development
- Students have clear goals in their training for future employment
- Educators design quality and focused instruction consistent with the needs of the industry
- Consumers enjoy high quality, efficient health care delivery by well-trained workers (National Health Care Skill Standards Project, n.d.).

Manpower training needs to be defined and implemented, whether within an individual organization or an entire health care system. The organization that tools up the skill capabilities of its people is equipping itself for success. It may use either outside reference points or devise a sensible internal approach. As a practical matter, health care organizations should not wait for full blown development of standards. Start now to intensify training, and make sure its coverage is in line with standards deemed acceptable by local professionals. Once a solid program is up and running, standards can be gradually increased and fine tuned.

The Destruction of Culture

Perhaps leadership's biggest failure has been the damage to the culture of health care organizations. Human values were dying under the onslaught of decisions focused too heavily on financial results. In the mid and late 1990s, a number of health care executives were accused of illegal financial manipulations in various kickback schemes and Medicare fraud. Columbia/HCA Healthcare Corporation became the most publicized example of what was occurring in many organizations and systems throughout the nation as promise outran performance. The creation of chains was beginning to result, not in the hoped for benefits, but in organizations that, if not out of control, were far from running smoothly. The financial gains supposed to result from a consolidation strategy were proving illusive as "savings" were being offset by defections, loss of morale, and huge increases in legal and liability problems.

As the pressures for expansion and profitability grew, an over-controlling dictation of operations ensued. This reduction of decision-making authority in some systems tended to further erode the historical buffer of local people serving local needs. That this inevitably led to reduced ethical standards and alleged illegal behavior was yet another betrayal of the common holy ground on which all of health care must be built. This sacred turf of ethics and values for service, respect, and excellence was often ripped by corporate greed and executive malpractice. The continuing stream of such stories brings to memory General Omar Bradley's condemnation of earlier business profiteers, whom he labeled "ethical infants, moral adolescents."

Today, health care workers in some organizations have far lower trust of management. They are more change resistant, and they turn to unions for representation against what they see as a leadership that will not protect their interests or the organization's. "Once stung, twice wary." This failure to protect the true interests of the organization, whether the jobs of the people or business reputation, all for the sake of short-term financial gain, was a frontal and violent attack on the health care industry's core values of caring, respect, and teamwork. This betrayal has created immense morale problems, complicating the task of the new leaders who instinctively realize the need to restore and repair this havoc. As Goethe noted well in *Hermann und Dorothea,* "For in these perilous times, the man whose mind is uncertain only spreads the evil wider and wider, while the man of firm purpose builds a world of his liking."

Culture has been described as the only lasting competitive advantage. Rosabeth Moss Kanter (1991) concluded in her studies of successful organizations that there are four areas of essential competitiveness, which form mantras of how to compete:

1. Core competencies: Get really good at the core skills and services and exploit these rather than dabbling in areas where competencies will always be marginal.
2. Time compression: Do what you do faster to meet market expectations and drive costs down.
3. Continuous improvement: The market doesn't want junk, keep moving standards up.
4. Relationships: This area includes customer relations, but focuses more on the web and weave of internal culture and connection with suppliers as part of a seamless team.

To maximize these sources fully, Kanter recommended paying more attention to human factors. She found that the ineffective use of these four competitive sources stemmed largely from internal, social problems rather than from external market or strategic barriers. Existing, rigid distinctions between organizational classes such as levels, functions, and structural divisions interfered with adaptive capability. Organizations must not only remove these social barriers (such as privileged parking spots and catered meals), but also cease maintaining distinctions between organizational classes on the basis of the individual's "need to know." (Correctives might be combining internal newsletters going to different publics, and publishing the strategic plan for all Associates to take home.)

Finally, in the kind of corporate culture that creates a truly *sustainable competitive advantage*, Kanter found that managements looked for entrepreneurial ideas less from external consultants and more through seeding and feeding numerous small ideas arising from staff in numerous experiments—a high use of intellectual capital in a culture that encourages its expression.

This was succinctly illustrated in a brilliant piece chronicling why information technology, though important and vital, does not represent a sustainable advantage. Wrote the interviewer, Geoffrey Colvin (1997):

No one expresses the particular power of a cultural advantage better than Herb Kelleher, founder and CEO of Southwest Airlines, famed for its strong culture of humor and individual responsibility.

Once—mostly to provoke him, I admit—I tried telling Herb that his culture wasn't all that important. "I can explain Southwest's success," I said. "You fly one type of aircraft, serve no meals, transfer no luggage, give no assigned seats, fly mostly short hauls, and always charge the lowest fares on your routes. There's the formula. What's culture got to do with it?" Perhaps steam didn't actually shoot out of his ears, but it looked as if it would. He slammed the table and said, "Culture has *everything* to do with it—because everything you said our competitors could copy tomorrow. But they can't copy the culture, and they know it." Actually some of his competitors, notably United on certain California routes, later tried to copy almost everything I mentioned. But Herb was right: They couldn't copy the culture and got beat. [Geoffrey Colvin, "The Changing Art of Becoming Unbeatable." Reprinted from the November 24, 1997 issue of *Fortune* by special permission; copyright 1997, Time Inc.]

The same article chronicled a Wharton study that looked at the returns of money invested in infotech (software and hardware) versus money invested in IT workers in the banking industry. The conclusion was that whereas capital investments "may be a strategic necessity to stay even with the competition," far greater returns were obtained from investments in the workers.

What Should Management Do with People?

Executives whose organizations win are invariably great as leaders of people. They understand the two greatest secrets of business: The toughest and most critical tasks have to do with people. If you can fill those needs, the people will handle all the other problems that beset the organization and go on to create and develop its business opportunities. So the prescriptions for raising standards in managing people are in two broad areas: first, create a great job environment that fires up the team; second, turn on the megavoltage of human ideation.

Restore the Workplace

It ought to be clear to even the most casual observer that you can't win with losers (management or staff), nor can you win with a mere of collection people who aren't a team. To build a business, you must start by building the people. Management must construct a work environment that attracts and retains talented people and that uses all that they have to give. Microsoft has done that, Disney has, and so has Southwest. How those organizations deal with their people isn't for warm or fuzzy reasons or out of mushy humanism, it is for hard business reasons. Though human values certainly are central in successful organizations, they are central because they're good for business.

What are the basics of good people management that must be created or redefined as the foundation for higher performance? What are some of the core elements and tasks that must be addressed to upgrade the performance levels of health care people at work? After all, if we are to heal others we must first heal ourselves (Sherman, forthcoming). Standards of health care will be dramatically improved when the organization gets the following basics right:

Select intensively. No more hiring "warm bodies," no more thinking "you have to take who you can get in a tight labor market." Multiple interviews, and multiple interviewers, have proven to improve substantially the quality of Associates working in high performance organizations. Given normal turnover, this can have a dramatic impact on the overall organizational mix in as little as a year or two. Remember: The best of workers can be as much as twice as productive as the least. Pay at least as much attention to attitude as skills. You can add to skills, but its almost impossible to change attitude.

Remove problem employees. In the Information Age the choice is either to retrain or replace people. Removing deadwood drag will help team after team function better. A small percentage of problem workers cannot be allowed to run the ranch. Marginal workers often realign their drift-along performance when they see that behavioral standards must be met (Sherman, 1987).

Redesign jobs. Make jobs bigger via cross training and increase the power of individuals and work teams. This usually is accomplished in conjunction with redesigning work processes but can also be achieved by combining small departments or stripping out excess layers of management. Having a powered-up work force depends on three critical support pieces: lots of training, information technology, and all the work tools people need to do the job.

Grow people. We are no longer interested in personnel administration or human resources management. Let's get the language right. These are people, not personnel or resources. It is their brains and spirit that can keep us competitive. Intense development as a focus is essential, as is the resultant multiskilled workforce. Training has a bonus: It gives people a sense of security (knowledge is power) and helps them understand the changing pattern of work processes. In this new age the ethic seems to be to promise *employability*: If you come with us we will keep your skills abreast should you decide to leave us.

Pay well. Stop the silly game of paying people the lowest wage possible. Lower wages do not equal lower labor costs. Pay people little, and they bring low gusto and productivity to the job. Strive to be in the top half of employers in regards to salary, the ideal spot is to be at the bottom of the top third. Paying top dollar isn't necessary if the organization offers the additional "paycheck" of "best place to work." Stop step increases, cost of living adjustments, overall organization performance incentives, and other killers of achievement. Put all salary dollars into merit and measurable individual and team incentives. Compress wages, have fewer levels and wider ranges. Deemphasize pay and worry over dollars. Add lots of socialization, recognition, celebration, and motivational events. People do not live by "bread" alone.

Retain winners. It's been said that loyalty is dead. Let others buy that drivel. If other employers don't show loyalty, and you do, you've just gained another competitive advantage. Unless health care is willing to commit to its staff, it cannot expect commitment in return or extra effort. *Retain the best.* Use retention profiles to help selected people stay with you—these are the ones that others like to discriminate against. Hire older workers, those with disabilities, working moms. Provide the support elements people need such as a day care center, remove work irritants, improve the quality of work life. Consider promising no layoffs after a certain number of years.

Restructure the organization. The organization is its people. Make the structure of the organization fit what works for the people. Usually that means fewer levels and fewer departments. It always means fewer status differentials—no privileged parking or catered meals. Executives have to ask themselves: Which do we want more—privileges or results? Remove remote-control management as a style; reduce the segregation between managers and Associates and between departments. A Jeffersonian egalitarianism is how Americans like their relationships.

Keep the Faith

A new philosophy is at work in America's organizations, based on an awareness that the toughest challenge in management is the people stuff. Ineffective executives fool themselves in thinking that what they do with product and pricing, finances and marketing, or multiunit-system design are the hard tasks. They have it backward. All that may be difficult, but it is secondary work and infinitely easier than building an on-fire culture. If creating a feisty team is so easy to do, why haven't they done it?

The 100 Best Companies to Work for in America identified organizations that had distinguished themselves as places to work. Updated several times since its original publication and reported annually in *Fortune*, the 1998 Honor Roll listed the following as the Top Ten and commented on their culture [R. Levering and M. Moskowitz, "The 100 Best Companies to Work for in America." Reprinted from the January 12, 1998 issue of *Fortune* by special permission; copyright 1997, Time Inc.]:

1. Southwest Airlines. A typical comment: "Working here is a truly unbelievable experience. They treat you with respect, pay you well, and empower you. They use your ideas to solve problems. I love going to work!"
2. Kingston Technology. Year-end bonuses averaged $75,000 per employee at this computer memory maker.
3. SAS Institute. This software company has on-site child care, a pianist plays in the cafeteria, and turnover is at 4 percent in an otherwise high-turnover industry.
4. Fel-Pro. This auto-gaskets maker focuses on employees' kids: $1000 savings bond at a child's birth, day care, summer camp and summer jobs for the kids, and $3500 college scholarships.
5. TD Industries. All of the stock of this Texas air conditioning company is owned by employees, who at monthly meetings decide how to run the business. "This company makes you feel like a human being again."

6. MBNA. Credit card issuer's No. 1 hiring criterion: "People who like other people."
7. W. L. Gore. Gore-Tex producer has dozens of "sponsors" to set the pace, doesn't have traditional organizational hierarchy and managers.
8. Microsoft. Every person gets stock options. Most professionals hired before 1992 have become millionaires. Bill (never Mr. Gates) personally answers all e-mail from employees.
9. Merck. The consistently best-performing pharmaceutical house, where the corporate credo is to put patients before profits. Thirty-one percent of managers are women.
10. Hewlett-Packard. "They walk the talk when they say their people are their most important asset." Recently added: domestic-partner and nursing home care for spouses, parents, and grandparents to an already fat benefit package.

It should come as no surprise that many of these same names appear on the list of *Fortune*'s "Most Admired Companies," whose business results lead all others in their industries. What was hypothesized only a few years ago—that there might be a correlation between excellence of work place and subsequent business performance—is now close to being proven, though some say it's a chicken-and-egg problem. Do high morale workers create profits or is it the other way around? Clearly running a business is more than just focusing on staff. You had better keep your eye on work processes and customers, too. Although there is a variety of piecemeal evidence to debate these points, a recent report from Ernst and Young found that institutional investors are now "more likely to buy stock on a company's ability to attract talented people. They're betting cash that it makes a difference" (Grant, 1998). Want to win? Create a winning team.

These ten winning best place to work companies averaged forty-one hours of training (versus an average of six hours in hospitals) and 6 percent turnover (often twice that at hospitals), statistics that most hospitals would love to have.[1] Though each of

---

[1] Other benchmarks of average training effort in corporate America in 1996: Training expenditures averaged 2.9 percent of payroll; $1526 of total training expenditure per employee; 175 employees per training staff person (American Society for Training and Development, n.d.).

these working environments were different, Gallup's survey of 55,000 workers attempted to match employee attitudes with business results and found four attitudes that, taken together, correlated strongly with higher profits: "Workers feel they are given the opportunity to do what they do best every day; they believe their opinions count; they sense that their fellow workers are committed to quality; and they've made a direct connection between their work and the company's mission" (Grant, 1998).

These findings make the point that the goal is not simply to make everybody feel good, or to return to the old paternalism. Rather, the goal is to create a higher order of consciousness: When work is important to the worker, individual effort is tied correctly into a supportive corporate culture that animates and energizes the attainment of business objectives.

It's one thing to be able to offer stock options if your company is a rocket, but what can organizations do who are fighting resource scarcity? At the annual Congress of the American College of Health Care Executives, I asked an audience of 500 how many of their organizations sent Associates a birthday card. Approximately 15 percent responded affirmatively. Yet sending birthday cards is the first thing Southwest talks to people about who visit them for benchmarking. If your eyes glaze over at such simple suggestions, you might not be able to comprehend the message that a lot of what works isn't costly. Identifying the key turn-ons can help management avoid wasting a lot of time and money on expensive benefits that produce almost no return to the business. *Fortune's* summation was that three characteristics seem to run through all the highly rated workplaces (Levering and Moskowitz, 1998):

1. Inspiring leadership. About Mary Kay Ash, founder of Mary Kay Cosmetics, it is said that not only does she inspire people to work hard and succeed, but she also motivates them to become like her—a woman who wants to create economic independence for other women. For her, her business was all about fulfilling a mission bigger than the job itself.
2. Knockout facilities. Buildings aren't important in themselves, but they can be critical in telling Associates that they're valued. (I encountered dirty crew rooms with broken furniture in one hospital recently.) Winning workplaces usually have impressive corporate compounds (typically with child care fa-

cilities), great food (so good it's ordered for takeout), athletic facilities and intramural leagues, playgrounds, and many occasions for picnics. These amenities can cost a lot, but they achieve a lot.

3. A sense of purpose. A fat bottom line is not worth giving your life for; health care organizations that forgot that are dropping like flies. Medtronic, an electronic device maker, has patients whose lives were saved by their product flown in, along with their families and doctors, to employee meetings to tell survival stories. Couldn't that be done in our health care organizations as well? It is time for the return of high-minded talk in health care. We are on a mission, and when our people know it and feel it, they will transform the organization around them.

Conclusion

This chapter has shown that business success comes from the people working in that business. In many health care organizations, leaders must repair the cultural damage, anxiety, and job insecurity created by layoffs and other poor decisions that betrayed core values of the enterprise. We have to move human management, job structures, rewards, and many other elements in new directions to create a superior workplace. Until that is done, all other curatives will at best be only partially successful. Viewing people as the drivers of change, and working on their concerns first, will produce successful outcomes for Customers and the organization. The establishment of a new human culture is the prerequisite to excellence. What needs to be done in your organization? Ask the people, individually and in surveys. Be prepared for an avalanche of suggestions, which is exactly what you need. In the next chapter we'll address the question of how to install best practices. But installing best practices and releasing intellectual capital are only made possible by having first fixed the work climate.

Work-Out Session

1. Start with the facts. What are the reasons for unwanted turnover, especially among employees you want to keep? What do opinion survey data identify as key issues disturbing Associates? If the data aren't available, get them.

2. What behavior deserves recognition but is being reward-starved? What new reinforcement schemes could be devised at a departmental level? At an organization level?
3. Training is a major prescription. What's needed in basic orientation, basic skills training? What about orientation to culture and values? Do people know how to solve problems in small groups?
4. Where are job parameters or expectations unclear? Where do people feel that they have little autonomy? Pick two to three jobs and redesign them to be more doable by real people. Ask the people in those jobs what they think is needed.
5. Is culture being damaged by bad hiring decisions or the continued presence of problem workers? What needs to be done to turn the workplace into a community of winners?
6. Are leaders spending enough time working on people needs and building the fire of human skill and commitment, or are they wasting time and effort fighting fires of things gone wrong?

Chapter Nine

Best Practices Make Perfect

We need to find better ways to do things in health care. For example, health care's cycle times and wait times are notorious. David Letterman reported that one patient had spent eight hours waiting in a hospital's emergency room, and finally went home to die of natural causes! He thought it was a joke, but commonly enough emergency room patients get so fed up with waiting that they do leave. What does it mean when the lines from the best gag writers in the business are actual descriptions of health care's work processes? Bob Newhart said he called his doctor's office for an appointment but they told him it would be a month before they could work him in. "I could be dead by then," Bob exclaimed, whereupon the receptionist said, "No problem. If your wife lets us know we'll cancel the appointment!"

We need to find better ways to do things, and we need to do it now. In this chapter we're going to navigate the ocean of best practices and benchmarking, and figure out how to import intellectual capital from outside the organization, as well as listen to best thinking internally.

Benchmarking is a simple concept. Find a current best practice happening in some other organization, figure out how to adapt it to your circumstance, implement it, and pray that results will be better than the old practice it replaces. Benchmarking usually provides at least incremental, sometimes phenomenal, improvement. As a change strategy it's a lot smarter than trying to continuously improve existing in-house processes, for it shows people how widely different the best practice is from what's been home grown, and it's a lot faster. Benchmarking is a key tool that should be used by every department and profession as standards move higher: Don't reinvent the wheel.

A problem that relates to this is the current lack of *best practice clearinghouses,* libraries from which much of this information could be drawn. This is a need that state, national, and professional groups must address. As I wrote this book I searched in vain for Internet clearinghouses sponsored by many of the health professions. This lack is a very real problem for those managing health systems and individual organizations who are having to duplicate invention every time they turn around. For twenty years I have done organization renewal work: Each hospital has always had to build from scratch. This chapter will provide some ideas and sources that may be useful in resolving this problem.

Defining Best Practices

The phrase *best practice* is a misnomer. There can never be a best practice in the ultimate sense of the phrase. Best practices might more accurately be defined as

- "Best heard of"—we're not aware of anything better
- "Best next step"—it's not ideal, but it's an improvement over present practice
- "Best belief"—no data, but we think it's the best thing around
- "Best for now"—today's greatest is tomorrow's obsolescence

Labeling something a best practice doesn't necessarily make it so. There are limits to what the phrase means. The American Productivity and Quality Center in Houston defines a best practice this way: "There is no single 'best practice' because best is not best for everyone. Every organization is different in some way—different missions, cultures, environments, and technologies. What is meant by 'best' are those practices that have been shown to produce superior results; selected by a systematic process; and judged as exemplary, good, or successfully demonstrated. Best practices are then adapted to fit a particular organization" (American Productivity and Quality Center, 1998).

In less technically or procedurally defined areas of work such as personnel or marketing, what passes for a best practice is what professionals in the field consider to be the best idea or procedure to date. There may be some research to support certain ideas as beneficial (for example, pay for performance) but not necessarily a specific technical approach. In such work arenas there will always be debate over whether one particular practice is better than another, but there will also be a strong consensus over what the better approaches are.

In science-derived areas like medicine or laboratory operations, there may still be insufficient certainty in the research, often because practitioners are operating on what is always an expanding edge of knowledge. Even in these work arenas there tends to emerge a consensus among physicians that one treatment approach, or a limited range of treatment options, are clearly better than others. Problems arise when that consensus falls behind what new research is showing.

Many hospital executives are aware of the best practices concept but have done little to take advantage of it. They still have the mindset of doing what others are doing, imitating rather than initiating a new approach. The mediocre copy the mediocre. But those who lead the industry into its future know that health care needs to get out of the box and start copying best practices in organizations *outside* the hospital industry.

Let's be clear. Best practices are not a fad. They are not here today, gone tomorrow. We embrace best practices as a constant target and recognize that approaches like continuous improvement, benchmarking, suggestion programs, and Customer surveys are only means to that goal. Nor are best practices limited to clinical processes or simply the domain of quality management. They cut across the total range of activities and are part of all that we do.

We're humble enough to recognize that as best practices are installed, they immediately begin to obsolesce. Nature, a best-practice system, teaches that all cells die and must be replaced with new cells. Whatever best practices we install, we know we eventually will have to replace them with newer thinking—hence the concepts of knowledge management, continuous improvement, and management's responsibility to add to the body of knowledge. Because we must be in the modality of forever replacing, we can be nondefensive about the status quo. We are creative destroyers, steadily creating the future and deliberately destroying the past to make way for it.

What Should Best Practices Cover?

The short answer to the question of how widespread best practice emulation should be in health care is that it should be found everywhere, in every practice and performance, in every department and every job. (Should less-than-best practices have any part of health care?) The reality, however, is that so much improvement is necessary that we need some plan as to where to start and how to proceed.

In some cases, best practices have largely been defined by the professions and simply need to be rigorously installed and people trained to follow them. Nursing tasks have been thoroughly studied and documented. One problem for nursing is job design, figuring out what a nurse assistant, LPN, or RN should do. That is, the profession's problem has more to do with authorities and appropriateness than how a task should be done and with training people in those defined procedures at the nurse assistant level. Yet nurse assistants are often trained in nonstandardized programs, and even licensed positions don't uniformly follow nursing procedures.

In other cases, there is some portion of a profession's work that has been defined, with other pieces still in flux. Here the task is to plug in what is agreed to, and make a judgment call on the rest. At the very least, remove some of the variability by picking one approach over the other when there are several acceptable avenues. One nursing director found that sterile dressing changes were being performed four different ways among her staff, and that not all were acceptable. Little differences like this can evolve into variations that can lead progressively downhill to infection and death. She picked the approach that was more correct and then asked for a standard curriculum to help standardize content in their refresher skills training.

Finally, where there are no standard definitions, assess the degree of business value and feasibility of setting some defined practices into place. Often this is an area in which substantial gain can be made over competitors; that is, there is no roughly equivalent response on their part if you move your organization forward in arenas of this kind. Example: An organization-wide, defined approach to how management should do its job.

Where Should Health Care Benchmark?

In the past, hospitals tended to mimic practices in other hospitals. This led to an improvement margin that was too narrow. The health care enterprise has been variously described as an incestuous cottage industry, an industry where everyone knows everyone, an old-boy, old-girl network, an enterprise imperiled by group-think. Although this state of affairs may feel cozy and even have certain advantages, it also contains the risk of thinking inside the box, closed off from the evolution of management theory and practice. Hospital executives have been described as migrants moving only within the confines of the industry, in contrast to immigrants coming from other industries. If the current state of the industry was better, perhaps this wouldn't be a problem.

An increasing number of hospital executives are requiring their organizations to think "outside the box." One exercise we've found useful with our clients has been to impose a year's moratorium from benchmarking on other hospitals, making exceptions as necessary. During this time unit leaders are required to benchmark quarterly outside the industry. The question they ask themselves isn't whether they're doing what other hospitals are doing, or whether they are the best in the hospital industry, but whether they are the best in the world in any industry. Not only does this approach force minds to rethink things, but it also assures that the benchmarking work will represent a greater leap—one more likely to delight Customers, improve quality, and affect ROI. GE CEO Jack Welch described this approach in a GE letter to shareholders (1997): "GE began to systematically roam the world, learning better ways of doing things from the world's best companies. . . . Our behavior is driven by a fundamental core belief: the desire, and the ability, of an organization to continuously learn from any source, anywhere, and to rapidly convert this learning into action is its ultimate competitive advantage."

Again, from the American Productivity and Quality Center (1998), benchmarking is "the process of identifying, learning, and adapting outstanding practices and processes from any organization, anywhere in the world, to help an organization improve its performance. . . . Benchmarking is action—discovering the specific practices responsible for high performance, understanding how these practices work, and adapting and applying them to your organization."

Ask yourself, "Who is more likely to have a better and more thoroughly tested approach to Customer relations, Disney or any hospital we know? Who is more likely to give us breakthrough ideas in materials management, Wal-Mart or any hospital we know? Who would be a better teacher in quality control, Motorola, which practices "perfection management," or any hospital we know?" Although a number of New American Hospitals have copied outside practices and may now be worthy of emulation, I still suggest going directly to the national or world leading organization and making your own adaptation. Adaptation is a problem, because creative thought and energy are required. But with creative involvement with best concepts come buy-in, commitment to new approaches, and high-quality solutions.

The Knowledge Management Problem

The list below shows the sequence of the birth of knowledge, its subsequent development to the point of usability, the problem of getting it accepted by those using older concepts, and finally its implementation as standard operating procedure. The central challenge for management is rapidly and everywhere to adopt new knowledge for the benefit of business and health care outcomes.

Steps to Implementing Knowledge

1. Hunches, hypothesis, and basic research. The creative mind is where knowledge is born in each profession and every department. Challenge: Are enough ideas being born, nurtured?
2. Knowledge evaluated and proved in the field. Solutions now exist. The process is the ongoing refinement of application. Challenge: Are new practices located and adopted early?

3. Professional acceptance of the practice. Endorsements are needed by the profession to establish a new idea as a best practice. Challenge: Communication with and resistance from those trained twenty years earlier.
4. Implemented as standard practice. Approved best practice is put in place. Challenge: Is management driving them in?

Health care has failed to meet the challenge of each of these four steps: First, management isn't listening to enough ideas in health care. Ideas, except those consultants are paid for, are not widely generated, gathered, or implemented. Second, ideas that are adopted often go untested, hence there's an 80 percent failure rate on total quality management (TQM), guest relations, and other ideas. (Often the idea is sound but it fails anyway.) Third, many health care professions, though they debate endlessly, fail to provide defined and endorsed protocols of practice. Finally, even when better ideas are known, management fails to push them into being. Knowledge must be managed into place, it doesn't just drift in or osmose through the walls. Timeliness and speed of implementation of best practices in the Information Age will spell the difference between those who win and those who lose.

Converting Knowledge into Action

A number of problems must be managed in bringing new knowledge into use in your department or organization in line with the steps outlined above. What can management do?

1. Insist on a set number of implemented suggestions for change per person on payroll. Foment a culture that welcomes ideas, provides mechanisms for training, and uses measures that assure that this intellectual capital will be seeded continuously in the organization.

2. The new standard of communication is instantaneous, the route is the Internet. Each health care profession's journals have become obsolete except as they document information already on the wire. Even the nation's newspapers have parallel versions in cyberspace. There used to be a lag time between discovery and implementation of information that could be blamed on problems in disseminating and distributing knowledge. But the era in which

scientific discoveries took years to be disseminated is over. Any new AIDS discovery today will be known by all researchers tonight. Nursing, lab, pharmacy and all other professionals need to be able to download the latest and greatest tools and information *now*. As one association executive said about this lag problem, "It's time to get shakin' and bakin'."

3. Each of the health professions has now become its own major barrier to adopting new thinking through resistance caused by ignorance or politics. New approaches that will keep practitioners abreast with the benefits of new knowledge are required. The amount of time professionals spend locked in committees debating practice changes that will speed benefits to the field must be reduced. Already physicians are being upstaged by patients who know about and are demanding new pharmaceuticals, tests, and surgical procedures before the practitioner can come up to speed. The FDA learned that AIDS patients need faster approval times—and that is a necessary prescription for all new professional knowledge.

4. Slow-to-adopt managements will become less of a problem with the passage of time. Effective leaders know that ideas lead to solutions, and solutions lead to organizational success. A management that does not aggressively adopt new ideas is a liability that no health care organization can afford. One of the advantages of competition and resource scarcity is that it impels adoption of best practices for the tremendous resource that they represent. Managements that are unable to manage knowledge will simply be out of a job.

How Is Benchmarking Done?

One way to get to best practices, and get there fast, is by way of benchmarking. Benchmarking is a process of comparing one's own performance against that of another organization. In its simplest form, this is done simply by reading about it or seeing it in operation, judging it worthy of adoption, then changing things back home. For many elements this procedure works just fine, but it lacks systemization. What might be done with benchmarking to extract maximum benefits? (For reference, see Camp, 1989; Balm, 1992; Codling, 1992; Watson, 1992; Zairi, n.d.; Bendell, Boulter, and Goodstadt, 1997; Camp, 1995.)

Sylvia Codling has written extensively on benchmarking as a tool to gain competitive advantage. Her approach is strategically focused and effectively simple. She notes that most organizations benchmark against their competitors; this can highlight potential strengths and weaknesses but can never be a basis for continuous improvement. Why? If you're only becoming as good as your competitors, you're not going to produce competitive advantage: You can play catch up, but you can't leapfrog. She notes (Codling, n.d.):

> In benchmarking, it is all too easy to become obsessed with figures. You should remember that today benchmarking is 90 percent process and only 10 percent metrics. *This means it must be strategic rather than tactical* [italics added]. Organizations should start by identifying their core competencies—those strategic business capabilities which provide their business advantage. From this, they will be able to focus on the key business processes that deliver those competencies, and identify the critical success factors and key enablers for those processes. These are the areas which should be measured and only now should the organization begin to think about metrics.

Codling argues for benchmarking targeted to core business processes and strategic objectives, not peripheral activity. And she demystifies benchmarking by calling it "no more than well applied common sense." She goes on to make the case that internal focus, whether to your own organization or your own industry, is a mistake (Codling, n.d.): "Process benchmarking . . . is the most effective means of ensuring the continuous improvement. While increasing awareness of what you do well, it identifies what needs to change and why. Process understanding leads to more effective management, helping you to identify and set credible targets. But most importantly, it makes you into an externally focused organization that is in a position to learn from and take advantage of the experience of others. It certainly beats sitting up the proverbial tree and hoping your competitors give up."

Benchmarking is better than continuous improvement as a departure point because instead of marginally improving what is a mile short of what's being done outside, we can "leap tall buildings in a single bound." From a cultural perspective, benchmarking jars people out of their complacency. The concept of the New American Hospital was originally designed to get people to look outside the insular hospital industry. Once you get people looking outside, their vision of your organization is never the same when they come back home. That alone is worth the plane ticket for a benchmarking visit.

The Benchmarking Process

A brief examination of how benchmarking is done would be useful in the context of understanding the tool better, for it's one that should be used widely.[1]

Scope
The objectives of benchmarking are to

- Identify competitive position and relative weaknesses
- Identify "best of breed" practices
- Gather ideas about how breakthrough improvements can be achieved
- Develop truly innovative approaches to process redesign
- Develop new techniques for improving quality, service, and efficiency
- Help change the mindset toward process improvement

Targets
The targets for benchmarking could be any aspect of business operations. As a priority it usually makes sense to start with what would make the most significant improvements for Customers and profitability. Customers might like improvements in quality, consistency of service, cycle time (speed), esthetics, responsiveness to requirements, and adaptability to special needs. Profitability would be enhanced if benchmarks could be established for waste, inventory levels, reduction of lost time, or staff turnover.

---

[1] For the discussion on the benchmarking process, I owe a debt of thanks to the folks at Top-ix Ltd. in England for their lucid outline "Business Process Benchmarking," available on the Internet at www.metabpr.com/ben-mark.

Don't waste time benchmarking small, marginal or nonstrategic processes.

Methodology

Benchmarking tends to proceed through the following steps (see Figure 9.1):

1. Identify the process or procedure to be benchmarked. This may be a Customer issue, a time-siphoning procedure, or some other issue important enough to draw somebody's attention. It should be one of significance to the business, where the time or effort is worth investing. (If it is related to a BHAG or values question, you can count on it being worth undertaking.)

2. Measure how well you're doing the process currently. This will represent the baseline against which improvement can be judged. Effective managers make this quantitative when possible, subjective when necessary. Thinking through how to recognize when you're making progress has positive payoffs down the line.

3. Identify who or what organization is best. Identification can be done by literature search, networking, or one's own observation. Usually there are a wide number of candidate organizations. Determining who is "best" to benchmark on should have some relevance to the kind of business practice one is comparing. Looking at Disney's people management practices might fit almost all work environments, but looking at how Ford makes cars might be more of a stretch in terms of making adaptations. Because the correct strategic market position for health care organizations is Operational Excellence, it would be best to benchmark on an organization pursuing the same strategy—highly efficient, low-cost, Customer-satisfying businesses such as Southwest Airlines, McDonald's, and Wal-Mart, as detailed in this book.

4. Find out how the benchmark organization does the task. Don't be concerned with why, and don't edit out the pieces you don't think fit. A common error is to edit out elements you think don't fit or apply before you understand what's going on. Be most concerned in understanding all the specifics, their sequence, support processes, and training. Take pictures, videos, and copious notes. It also might be a good idea to take a whole team with you to be really sure you get the picture. If Julia Child is teaching you

Figure 9.1. The Benchmarking Improvement Cycle.

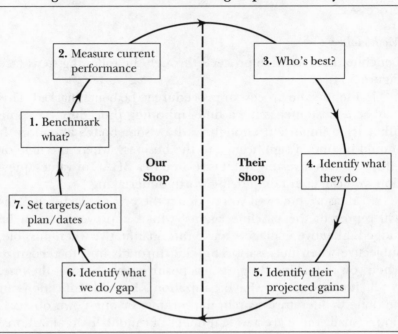

her best recipe, you would be smart to write down everything you're told, and then do every little step, including the ones you don't understand. If Julia is benchmarking you, you no longer need to take notes.

5. Determine where the benchmark is trending. It's also a good idea to find out where your benchmarking partner is going. It's highly likely that a benchmark organization isn't going to stay where they are, and it would be a mistake to set the benchmark at their current levels when they plan a 50 percent improvement in ninety days.

6. Look at how you're doing things back home. What are the step-by-step differences? How big is the performance gap? What accounts for this? What training, tools, practice differences will have to be introduced? What emerges as the probable causes of success in the outside benchmark?

7. Create and carry out an action plan. Make plans to make

change. What is to be changed? Who is in charge? When will it happen? What support will be needed?

As an example of benchmarking in practice, let's look at a non–health care example. (Think outside the box, right?)

Copy Rank Xerox

Rank Xerox is a $4.5 billion subsidiary of Xerox and sells copiers and document processors in Europe. Benchmarking has long been a deeply held belief within the corporation. Like most organizations, it is usually applied to the cost side of operations. What makes this example interesting, reported in *Fortune* ("Beat the Budget and Astound Your CFO," 1996), is that Rank Xerox decided to apply the technique to the revenue side of the ledger. The first step was to assemble a team of a couple of dozen people from various sales, service, and administrative staffs. The mission was to help divisions learn from each other throughout Europe.

In a matter of a few weeks they had assembled all kinds of sales data, doing a country-by-country comparison. They quickly found eight cases in which one country or another was dramatically outperforming all others; for example, France sold five times more color copiers than all other countries, Austria had only a 4 percent attrition rate on contract renewals whereas some countries had as much as 15 percent.

The next step was to send team members to the benchmark country. Their hard directive was simply to find out how it was done: Don't try to figure out how it worked. Once this was determined the team assembled a book for each country's sales and service managers (the people who could make change happen) that showed each benchmark and how that performer's system worked.

BEWARE THE SINKING ROCKS

Think about what was being attempted. The team was trying to ship in great new ideas to areas of the corporation that weren't using them. This is always an adventure in change resistance. Good ideas usually run aground on three rocks during the implementation phase. The team had to figure out a way around these rocks:

1. Data denial: "It just ain't so."

2. Exceptionalism: "Our market is different."

3. You can lead a horse to water, but you can't make him drink: "Your suggestions deserve careful study."

Denial wouldn't work because the team's documentation was not just about process but results—the benchmarks were clearly producing more. One of the reasons that separate divisions had been established was precisely because the organization wanted to encourage creativity. Yet this autonomy acted to undercut the transfer of best practice ideas in from other countries. The team decided to skirt these last two rocks by finding ways for people to save face and by providing a mixture of carrots and sticks:

• No country was the benchmark for more than one practice, so most areas got to teach as well as learn.
• Each country's team was told to pick three or four best practices, so they had the freedom to decide what would help their organization the most.
• Ambitious goals were set: Each country had to achieve 70 percent of the benchmark standard in the first year. That meant that going slow wasn't an option.
• One aspect of the change was mandated. There could be absolutely no changes in year one. This was meant to prevent people thinking that they could improve on the benchmark by fiddling with it, thereby ruining the very thing that made it work. In this case the watchword was, Don't think, just do.

RESULTS

Results were astonishing. Looking only at the best practices affected, and making sure there were no other causal factors at work, they concluded that year one sales increased by $64 million (1.4 percent of sales), year two by $200 million (3.64 percent). (Note: Lest the reader not understand the significance of these numbers, ask your CFO to plug those sales increases in on the revenue line of your organization's budget and watch his reaction when he hits Enter.)

Rank Xerox says there are a couple of obvious lessons here: There's clearly a lot of know-how lying fallow in the organization. If you can put it to good use it can make you a lot of relatively easy money, make Customers happy, and improve operations. The second lesson is that exceptionalism is the exception. It can be a real shock to people to find out that their unit or hospital is no different from any other, even though everyone initially thinks it is.

So get the data, identify the targets for improvement, and figure out a way to deal with the rocks.

Benefits of Benchmarking

The benefits of benchmarking include

- Getting people to think outside the box and outside the industry invariably leading to more creative solutions through the use of tested and proven solutions
- Forcing a reexamination of the way things are done now and kicking the organization out of its "comfort zone"
- Preventing people from reinventing the wheel in a period of scarce resources; saving time and cost when others have done it already, often better, cheaper, and faster
- Speeding up change and making implementation easier because of involvement and buy-in from those who work on the process
- Overcoming inertia and complacency with the status quo as people see the gaps revealed between current performance and the way it's being done elsewhere

The Best Practice Tool Shop

Space limits won't permit a full description of other tools and methodologies that can assist the achiever of excellence to install best practices, but a brief description of some of the more interesting approaches is in order. For the person new to installing best practices, the new terminology can at first seem confusing.

I remember visiting my father's small electronics plant when I was a boy. The test meters, oscilloscopes, lathes, and metal-fabricating machinery were fascinating to me, though I could only guess what each did. Al was my dad's chief technician. He was highly skilled and knew how to do everything. I began to understand that there was no magic to doing any of the tasks, but one did have to learn how to use the equipment. It was simply a learning curve problem. So, here's a quick orientation to what's in the best practices shop in the way of useful tools. Remember the following basic rules for learning to use the tools in this shop:

- None of this is rocket science. It's simply an organized way to identify work process elements and organize them into a better array to produce better outcomes.
- Don't use all the tools. Just use the ones that serve your purpose. You are the craftsman: The tools serve you, not the other way around. Following defined continuous improvement (CI) process might be the right approach to solving a need for improvement, but it also might be using the *Titanic* when a tugboat would do. Don't get hung up on process—think it through: What's the easiest way to solve this problem?
- Don't get fogged. Each tool is used either to help organize data to serve as a basis for discussion in problem solving or to help in documenting what will become the new practice and protocol. Nearly all people achieve their ends by making a picture of the process to assist visualization (85 percent of adult learning is through the use of the eyes—always make a picture).

Project Management Tools

Project management and continuous improvement tools include

- Gantt chart. Shows who does what when, and is useful when there are many pieces or people involved with a project.
- Cycle time reduction. Identifies the steps in a work process, travel distances, and time for each step. Helps to identify unnecessary steps, traveling, and waits.
- Work traffic diagram. Shows where people have to move in getting a job done.
- Histogram. Illustrates how much of something is happening per time unit over time.
- Control chart. Calculates how much variance is occurring and helps determine whether a work process is functioning normally or is out of control.
- Run chart. Shows variation in how much is happening and when but can't tell whether it's in the normal range (control chart junior).

- Pareto chart. Identifies the causes of a problem that represent most of it (80 percent) so that you're taking care of the baby whales instead of spoon feeding guppies.
- Flow chart. Shows step by step what task occurs before the next task in a work process. Different symbols are used as shorthand to symbolize the kind of work being done.
- Critical paths. Targets the most important tasks, those critical to the outcome of a work process or that are time-critical in that they must be completed before the next task can be done. As a tool, its greatest value would be for complex work processes, such as patient care work. It is a natural second stage after beginning with benchmarking. Critical paths may be overkill and not needed for simpler processes.

Health care has a few variations and additions to tools, such as clinical protocols, clinical pathways, care maps, and practice parameters. These are largely variations of flow-charting, critical paths, or defined work processes. Don't get lost in the fog of competing labels. Whatever the label in vogue is, ask whether it nails down what the defined best practice is. Are people then trained in that approach, and do measures show that it's working? Remember, best thinking cares less for tools and more for results. Tools are important only if they help people make change, and they do not have to be used in every case. Don't worship the tool, don't make any approach a religion.

Some organizations do not suffer from the "not invented here" syndrome, resisting ideas from outside. Their view of clinical paths and other defined clinical work processes is that they would rather trade dollars for time, and are willing to buy defined approaches from the many commercial services offering these in prepackaged format. Eventually, as we define our way through the backlog of undefined work processes and face only new processes and refining of old ones, the predominant course will be simply to import the processes and tweak them, focusing more of the internal effort on training how to do them and measuring outcomes. That is a preferable course when using organizations can be sure that the guidelines are reliable.

Along that line, HCIA has invited winners of its Top 100 Hospitals award to participate in clinical studies in an effort to organize a new database called the Clinical Benchmarks for Success. As reported in *Modern Healthcare,* this would be the "first national research database stratified by size and type of hospital and established solely on the basis of managerial and clinical performance" ("HCIA Launches Hospital Database," 1998). These steps would enable hospital managers to move quickly to take advantage of the tools such information provides.

Forward-thinking organizations aren't waiting for the benefits of a nationally defined set of best practice clinical protocols but are moving forward now to create them. One example is Memorial Health Services in Long Beach, California, which comprises five hospitals with 1,400 beds. Since 1993 the system has been searching for benchmarks, using clinical guidelines developed by interdisciplinary teams, and providing report cards to their communities. A key ingredient has been to standardize care procedures across the continuum of care so that the patient experience with specific tasks is the same whether in the hospital, at home, or in the physician's office ("In Search of Evidence," 1998). The importance of this effort is that the standardization on best practices has produced both better quality and cost outcomes. For example, the system reports that two radiologists read each mammogram, a cost picture that has proven less expensive than one reading because of fewer errors.

Other efforts are well along to further the dramatic gains possible with evidence-based medicine. The University of Pennsylvania Health System began in 1995 to define desired clinical outcomes and the standardized protocols that are required to reach them. They noted that variety in practice was leading to poor quality outcomes and increasing the cost of care. One of the distinguishing elements that made this more than the usual disease management program was that they established stretch goals to move rapidly across the entire system: By the year 2002, 80 percent of patient visits will be managed by these protocols. To reach that goal the organization is attempting to put ten more disease management programs in place per year to add to its existing defined knowledge base ("System Follows Protocol to Fight Disease," 1998). As in other systems wrestling with this problem, movement toward evidence-based medicine inevitably points out the need for evidence-based management. Variations in management practices, such as nonstandardized patient records, computer systems, and employee benefits, create tremendous costs, the dimension of which can only be guessed at, and are barriers to the implementation of clinical protocols—hence the argument for seeing standardization as a universal issue that affects all departments and work elements.

The problem of variation in clinical practice is a major driver of nonstandardization. Health care organizations largely respond to what physicians order up, so any effort toward standardization has to look upstream at both physician practice and education, and this reflects heavy interest now being shown among practitioners to defining best medical practices.

The *Journal of the American Medical Association* (D. Moore, 1998c) reported another disturbing aspect of variation in medical practice—the long lag time between discovery of a new treatment and its subsequent utilization. This "trickle down" problem was illustrated in a report on the use of beta blockers, which can significantly reduce illness and death in heart attack victims. Although these effects were known in 1982, beta blockers were being used on only 68 to 77 percent of "ideal" patients in five states in 1998. The other forty-five states were using the drugs on lower percentages of suitable patients, with the distribution falling to 30 to 38 percent in the five lowest states (D. Moore, 1998c). The National Committee for Quality Assurance made beta blockers a data element in HEDIS in 1996, having learned that what gets measured gets done, with subsequent raises in usage resulting. Although the work to be done is immense, the path is clear: Provide rapid communication to practitioners of research findings that have been digested enough to result in a recommended guideline, provide measures of outcomes, provide reeducation opportunities to come up to speed with the new procedures, and set some reasonable outside time limit by which practitioners must be following the better evidence-based approach.

There is an oft expressed view that healing is both a science and an art. We are now at a point of knowledge development where health care needs to become more science and less art in its practice. A report issued by Milliman & Robertson on guidelines for optimal hospital stays determined that 54 percent of "all in-patient hospital days . . . were medically unnecessary for commercially insured patients under the age of 65. For Medicare beneficiaries, that figure was 53 percent" (Kertesz, 1998). The report found significant regional variations in how physicians practice and how hospitals treat similar patients. "In most areas, a significant portion of providers were doing their business the way they want to—without rhyme or reason," David Axene, one of the firm's partners, reported. This variation in practice illustrates that too much "art" comes at a terrific cost. As knowledge builds, areas of fuzziness retreat. Defining best practice protocols leads to best results and sweeps away what are sometimes only best efforts.

Sources of Best Practices

There are lots of ideas and experimentation going on in health care. It is a wonderful time to change all kinds of things. But where can the best thinking be found, and how should we proceed to make the changes our health organizations need to make?

Professional Societies and University Programs

Historically the health care industry has looked to researchers, universities, and other knowledge manufacturers. But we don't want something academic or theoretical, we want the output of that earlier, upstream work. Organizations that deliver health care need results now. Nursing societies, and the voice of professionals in other occupations, then need to put their imprimaturs on the practices they accept. This endorsement is an important seal of approval, a needed component for the practitioner to have as a reliable guide. Individual hospitals, even systems, do not have the time or resources to do what the academic and professional groups must do.

In researching this book, I was able to find only a few best practice libraries sponsored by professional organizations. Best practices are either assumed to be known generally to the profession or are accessible in some other way. In an era of instant information flow, each professional group should publish on the Internet what the current state of the art is for their specialty, a clearinghouse of best practices that all can access. In cyberspace this can be housed anywhere, but in my view should be under the sponsorship of both the professional association and its university research sources. The day when health care tasks are not blessed by the profession is over. The lack of an authoritative source for proper practice, when people are nevertheless held legally responsible, is a recipe for disaster. Those who lead in pharmacy, nursing, and all other professions must push their association representatives and university sources for a clear, consistent statement of professional practice for each task and procedure. In this age, when all work processes are being defined with exactitude, to be silent on this question is a dereliction of duty.

Publishing and Consulting Houses

Publishers sometimes have to come to grips with the absence of articulation of professional standards by seeking a consensus from a panel of experts. For the delivery organization in the field, such texts may generally serve as an interim definitional standard. One effective nursing executive simply declared that procedures as outlined in *Lippincott's Manual of Nursing Practice* would be the basis for all in-house training and practice, thereby wiping out a wide range of practice variance and gaining greater control of operations in the process.

A number of consulting houses are now advertising best practice manuals, catalogs, and software. Most consultants (*consultant:* "a traveling textbook with frequent flyer miles"), ourselves included, have built files of stuff they've gathered in the field or had to create for past clients. Often these compendiums are useful little treasure chests that represent good platforms on which to build. It must also be said that calling something a best practice doesn't make it so, so *caveat emptor*.

Vendors and Contractors

When hospitals contract with Marriott to do food service, or with ServiceMaster to do housekeeping, what they're really buying are a set of benchmark practices that have already been field tested and have undergone serious continuous improvement efforts necessary to survive in their respective competitive industries. None of what they bring to the table couldn't be figured out in-house if you had twenty years to gain the experience and in-house expertise to solve the problem.

By defining themselves as a Customer service business, it was easy for McDonald's to outsource all of their distribution work and most other non-restaurant duties. Their suppliers provide the expertise on distribution, trucking, and warehouse best practices. McDonald's stays focused on Customer service, running the stands, and setting the tight, tough standards by which the outsourced work is controlled.

For hospitals, the lesson is clear: Copy internally the best practices that directly affect patient care, and do this by benchmarking outside the organization, even outside the industry; consider outsourcing for much of the other nonpatient care work *if* it can be controlled with tight standards from the hospital organization.

An annual vendors conference is another way to benefit from outside thinking. Invite staff from contractors to present their opinions on the directions they think the future will take and to present the tools and best thinking they have that could benefit what you do. Make it clear that the agenda is not a selling opportunity.

National or Regional System Libraries

As health care chains continue their consolidation, a number of them are beginning to create internal libraries of "plug and play" pieces (off-the-the-shelf programs and procedures) that can be used by their members. If you're in a system and this resource is available, use it. If your system hasn't started this idea, you ought to start it. In the competitive world faced by many health care systems there is clearly an advantage to being able to provide best practice services (one can almost hear the advertising campaign). But in addition to the powerful image of a provider whose quality and correctness is beyond peer goes the other business prize of lower cost.

If a movement toward national health care best practices does not materialize soon, system executives would be wise to aggressively seize the competitive opportunity and make the most of it. In the absence of a national approach, the power of using intellectual capital as competitive weapon will most assuredly follow.

Beware those who pursue standardization, for to these victors will belong the spoils.

The Problems of In-House Design

Best practices can be designed in-house but face a number of drawbacks. Local health care organizations often don't have either the staff time or expertise to design better approaches. They certainly have the intelligence, and many have worked, as we have, in hospitals across America. From a changing management perspective, however, we are rapidly reaching the end of the road where we have to invent something because no one else has thought of it. The answers are often available, and we're all short on time.

Inevitably when trying to make the decision of how to handle a project in a new knowledge area, management has to make a decision whether to *make or buy*. If your organization decides to *make* its best practice guidelines, greater buy-in is usually achieved along with a greater degree of custom fit, and this course is often politically more acceptable. If you *buy*, the purchase price is often offset by savings in labor cost and time that can be devoted to other projects. A purchased solution may still need some customizing, but at least you're starting with a standard recipe. One problem: How do we know what we're buying is really a best practice? The decision of which course to pursue may rest on how fast you need these practices in order to be competitive. A mix of both approaches may be possible: Make best practice guidelines in areas that are politically hot, buy them in areas that aren't. One idea is for each department to identify practices they want to change, then decide which to make, which to buy.

The Internet Treasure Trove

One of the prime values of the Internet is its ability to find newly born information and ideas. The Internet is growing in size at an exponential rate; 1997 estimates are over ten million addresses, a number expected to climb to over 200 million by the turn of the century. Truly a godsend for finding and evaluating best practice ideas, this powerful worldwide data system makes finding a large part of the accomplished pieces that can be used to elevate your organization doable. (Appendix B contains a list of sites related to standards and standardization.)

Use of a search engine, entering descriptors for best practices, benchmarking, clinical protocols, or continuous improvement, will pull up a long list of places to get started. It will also demonstrate the holes that still exist where some professions have not yet put this material on line or have not yet reached a consensus of best practices to recommend. If your profession is one of these, your recommendation for change may help push things along. You may also find only partial coverage of the procedures for which you need guidelines. We will soon be able to gain this information simply by dialing and downloading.

Best Practice Clearinghouses

The best source of help, when available, is from clearinghouses of best practices. These are becoming accessible at web sites where it is possible to fully offer a complete listing of items fitting a particular professional or topical area. When sponsored by a professional association, they carry the additional value of an endorsement on their offerings. One of the newer examples is the establishment by the Veterans Administration of an Information Resources Center (VIREC), which will centralize knowledge about all research projects and the 150 separate databases that are part of the VA system (J. Moore, 1998b). This will allow a clearer understanding of patient demographics, diagnostic information, admissions and discharge data, and the procedures and prescriptions involved in their treatment.

Another good example is an initiative led by the Massachusetts Hospital Association (MHA) to identify best practices in areas such as ordering and administering medication, and avoiding surgical mistakes. The MHA is working with the Massachusetts Coalition for the Prevention of Medical Errors. This group represents regulators, trade groups, doctors and nurses, and others to gather, evaluate, and disseminate information. Their vision is then to make adaptations for other settings, such as nursing homes (Morrissey, 1998c).

There is a need to cluster all health care practices in one or more such clearinghouses. These focused libraries not only would save a great deal of time and effort, but would also allow a greater ability to do side-by-side analysis of competing ideas. For now, however, you will need to find stuff where you can. As more focused libraries emerge they will materially affect the quality of care in America.

National health associations might choose to take the lead in such a best practices project for the benefit of their members. Certainly their reputation and clout make them candidates for this leadership role. Dr. Susan Adelman, a member of the American Medical Association House of Delegates, proposed that the AMA sponsor a clearinghouse for critical pathways. A version of that idea has now become reality, with peer reviewed guidelines for practice published at the AMA's web site (www.ama-assn.org). Her expression of the problem applies equally well for other health care professions. Translate it into what would make implementation of best practices easier for your own profession.

For a number of years the AMA struggled with *practice parameters,* collecting them and packaging them. Typically these had been produced by one of the national specialty societies or by governmental agencies. Parameters had been based on extensive research and surveys of the literature. Dr. Adelman noted, however, that *clinical pathways* were often being assembled by a small group of doctors in a hospital department who wrote out what they thought was the most cost-effective antibiotic regime for ruptured appendicitis or when a nasogastric tube should be removed. She noted that pathways just appear, gain local consensus, and are changed if local people have problems using them. The first approach is methodical, slow, and endorsed; the second is guided by trained professionals who are trying new concepts, is fast, and handles today's question, "How should I do this?" The AMA was publishing practice parameters, but Dr. Adelman asked, "What about pathways?"

> For one thing, pathways are proliferating like ants, are highly ad hoc, are not necessarily authenticated, and are completely unstandardized. On the other hand, they seem to work. *Unfortunately, most of our members are reinventing the same wheel simultaneously all over the country in their respective hospitals and health plans* [italics added]. For starters, they have to pick a format—that is, if they cannot copy

one from their hospital across the city. Then they create protocols within each category, unless they can find something to imitate. In short, we are all doing what we did several years ago when we wrote utilization programs, grievance processes, credentialing processes, and contract review processes for our health care plans. We copy someone else.

Then she suggests that the profession set up a best practice clearinghouse for these emerging pathways:

It would seem more practical and sensible for the AMA to set up an electronic bulletin board for members to post their current pathways for common conditions, operations, and illnesses. Obviously the AMA would need a disclaimer a mile wide and as high as the screen assuring the reader that the AMA does not endorse any of these pathways. Still, seeing examples of multiple pathways would be enormously helpful to those of our colleagues who are starting at point zero all over the country. They at least would have starting points, ready for local variations.

The arguments against pathways are the same as those against parameters. They are cookbooks, may be a liability risk, may not be valid, insult the expertise of physicians who do not need them, give too much information to nonphysicians, and so forth. For the sake of simplicity, I will concede all of these objections, to some extent. Nevertheless, pathways are being written and used. They also may prove to be an essential foundation for outcomes assessment. The job of the AMA in the areas of quality measurement and cost containment is to help its members help themselves. If members are using pathways in these efforts, we should make it easier for them. If pathways help them format outcomes assessment studies, we should support pathways. If they turn out to be the key to successful outcomes assessment, AMA will be in on the ground floor, and can take credit for them. [S. H. Adelman, M.D., "A Proposed New Clearinghouse for Critical Pathways," www.msms.org/adelman/sa-8.htm. Used by permission of author.]

It is essential to understand that both avenues lead to progress within each profession. Think of parameters (defined clinical protocols) as derived by looking back at past history and data, whereas pathways are reasonable, best practice calls being made in the present. Although we are not as sure of our footing with pathways, eventually the research will turn them into parameters. The physician's problem has its parallel in other health care professions as well: People need answers we don't formally have. What should we do or attempt as a reasonable leap from what we know for certain?

Other professions also need to standardize formats and communicate existing best practices or pathways. Any practice so endorsed, in some prudent, conditional way, serves as a target, a target either to be achieved or to be surpassed with a newer, better approach. In essence each profession hangs out a sign that says, "This is the best approach we know of—does anybody have any better ideas?" The amount of time, work, and effort this would save each profession is incalculable, the benefit immense. The professions who choose to lead the health care revolution will want to join with the AMA in providing this essential communication.

Commercial services such as Physicians' Online (www.po.com) and others are beginning to offer similar data sources. In doing the research for this book I found numerous web sites regarding medical practice guidelines and protocols. Although it seems that all health professions have an Internet presence, nonphysician sites often seem limited to general information, policy statements, and job opportunities. At the time of this writing, few were found to have specific endorsed practice guidelines on line, though to do so is a natural progression, a needed next step. It would be helpful if each professional would push this issue into the forefront of discussion among peers and associations.

A National Health Care Best Practices Clearinghouse

As an industry vital to the nation's health and its future, health care needs to assemble a new edifice, a place in cyberspace where one can go to retrieve best practices easily for all types of health care work. This would serve as a national clearinghouse, a one-stop shop where any hospital department, health care profession, or service line can go for up-to-the-minute guides on implementing best practices.

When I began writing this book, the idea of a national clearinghouse was a dream. By the time I was halfway through, it was becoming a reality. In 1998, the National Guidelines Clearinghouse (NGC) came online (www.guideline.gov). It intends to make available a full range of current guidance on treatments for specific medical conditions. The NCG is a joint project among the federal Agency for Health Care Policy Research, the American Medical Association, and the American Association of Health Plans. The AHCPR has already produced a number of clinical practice guidelines that have been widely used and adopted. As practice guidelines proliferate elsewhere there needs to be a coordinating and testing operation to reduce duplication and provide critical review.

Anyone with a computer will be able to access clinical practice guidelines from the NGC, which will offer a wide selection of guidelines from public and private organizations. All health professionals will want to be involved in or linked to this project.

According to AHCPR, the rapid growth in guidelines, and the rapid changes evolving within them, were causing problems for end users. Differences in development and content further complicated their use. According to an AHCPR press release (Agency for Health Care Policy Research, 1997), the web site is supposed to

- Contain standardized information for thousands of guidelines such as title, sponsoring organization, author(s), and methodology used
- Provide guideline abstracts and, where possible, the full text of guidelines
- Compare and contrast the recommendations of guidelines on similar topics, with summaries covering major areas of agreement and disagreement
- Have topic-specific electronic mailing lists to enable registered users to communicate with one another on guideline development, dissemination, implementation, and use

Both the AMA and the AAHP are strongly encouraging members who have been developing guidelines or databases to join with the effort to create the NCG, and it is anticipated that the large volume of work currently existent will speed the process of identifying effective practice outcomes. Currently the site doesn't rank or recommend one guideline over another.

How well the NGC accomplishes its task remains to be seen, but there's no question that this is the right road. That became increasingly evident when the call went out to one and all to submit any clinical practice guidelines for inclusion in the NGC database. The invitation in the *Federal Register* signaled that this would not be an exclusionary process, but one in which all professions can speak. Although this is currently in a physician-focused guideline database, it is clear that it will have a physician-driven impact on nonphysician practices in other health care professions; that is, it will be essential that other professions integrate their practice procedures in a complementary way. Inclusion criteria for submitted guidelines are rigorous but reasonable ("AHCPR Invites Clinical Practice Guidelines for Public/Private National Guideline Clearinghouse," April 13, 1998, press release). It is hoped that the NGC will be a source for the future, an example of the clustering and centralizing of best practice information.

An Approach to Best Practices Implementation

Regardless of what develops on the national scene, health care management's fundamental challenge remains, How can I implement best practices in my shop? Here's a short action plan of how this might be done:

1. Commit to a program of best practices implementation in all areas of your responsibility.
2. Set up a rapid-attack task group to organize a general plan of attack, set some dates for partial and complete implementation, and formulate some measures.
3. Identify existing sources of best practices *within the industry*—these are competitive benchmarks. Professional associations should be asked where their library of such practices is contained. If they don't have one, tell them to get on the bandwagon. Other sources are university researchers, books and publications, word-of-mouth networking.
4. Identify sources *outside* the industry. These are often, if findable, higher than health care industry benchmarks. Make sure you include some nontraditional sources in each departmental plan. Examine the question of whether to make or buy

when commercially available products are available. If consultants are used, keep them in advisory roles. Don't deny the achievement opportunity to your people.

5. Gather up improvement suggestions *inside* the organization. This is the most accessible source of ideation, has the greatest volume, is most quickly obtained, and has the greatest degree of buy-in. The key is to make sure that mechanisms for training and change support are in place before you ask for them, since a high implementation rate, quickly, is what is required. In our work we have sought ideas from these constituencies in this general overlapping order:

Managers. Their ideas include policy and procedure issues and remove these stumbling blocks for what is to come.

Associates. Sources of a huge volume of ideas that cover every room in the facility, every form, every patient interaction. They have clinical, nonclinical, and administrative suggestions.

Physicians. We've found that when they first see others actually making change, they become more willing participants. A majority of their suggestions tend to be clinical and Customer oriented. We usually work first on irritation removal for them, then move to the defining of clinical protocols that will affect many other work processes.

Customers. Patient issues first, then friends and family. Usually ideas are lightly solicited from them directly in the first year due to the volume coming in from the earlier sources, many of which directly affect Customers. This becomes more of a focused source in year two.

Suppliers. Vendors conferences or putting suppliers on project teams is a way to gain what is in essence a free consultancy.

6. Assemble a list of items to be changed. Push people's thinking. Is this going to be adequate to the task? Does it cover a wide enough area of operations? Is it getting at core business and Customer issues? Start to assess whether the changes you anticipate are a true best practice as indicated by hard research or endorsement by a profession, or whether the change is just an improvement, a better practice than what is now being

done. Accept both readily, but realize that some may leave a greater gap in improvement in the future that will need to be revisited.

7. Get started. This is the most important element. Use Do It Groups (DIGs) and Just Do Its (JDIs) and push for results. Don't forget to recognize and reward. Don't fail to celebrate each step in the marathon.

8. Create a general work plan, maybe a Gantt chart. The ongoing business is always a tumultuous situation, and you're having to make change at the same time that you have all your regular work to do. Keep reminding yourself, "Each improvement makes my load in the future easier." Remember, you're working yourself out of a hole. Each improved practice implemented means that you stop doing the old practice that took 50 percent longer or cost twice as much. Things *are* getting better.

9. Look again at the measures. Some will need to be refined or added, others will be dropped. If things are improving, the measures will show it. If not, keep changing until they do.

10. Keep your selling shoes on. Change creates questions and you must evangelize the good news of your progress.

11. Don't get discouraged. Not everything you try will work, but most things will.

12. If you're in a system, work to spread the good news of your success for other units that may want to borrow your ideas. You can then leapfrog them in the next round of competition.

Conclusion

This chapter has made the argument for the installation of best practices in all aspects of operations. Nothing less than that represents the values or mission of health care. Where possible, start by benchmarking to gain quicker and further progress. While the nation is beginning to gear up to better define and distribute best practices, early adopters will have an opportunity to outdistance both their own track records and their competitors.

In the concluding part of the book we will focus on the problems of managing change in order to achieve standardization of best practices. We'll begin in Chapter Ten by looking at the difficulties of making change in system organizations, as well as other organizational complications, and show how to avoid traps in change management to achieve the victory of a successful implementation.

Work-Out Session

1. Decide whether your department/organization should pursue and attain best practices status. Talk this up with staff, get people excited, sense who does and doesn't want to make the journey to excellence.
2. Sign a statement of commitment to excellence. "We, the people, have committed ourselves to making this the best admitting department of any hospital in the United States, and will accept nothing less." Make a big sign. Have everybody sign it. Post it where it's seen. Put yourself on the line.
3. Executives need to make the larger decision of whether they want all departments on a best practices footing. Assuming they do, what priorities among departments need to be set? Create a prioritized work list by department.
4. Get some common training going, circulate articles, find a few eager beaver managers to jump into the water first. Celebrate early and partial victories: Rome wasn't built in a day, but one day someone started to build it. Follow the benchmarking process in this chapter, or go on a best practices scavenger hunt.
5. Push for lots of small wins. The evidence in change management is that a ton of small wins is often more effective in galvanizing the organization than a few major changes.
6. Have fun! You're relentlessly pursuing excellence.

Part Four

Change Managing the Standardization Process

Behold, I make all things new.
—REVELATIONS 1:5

The work of organizational change is immensely challenging and tiring, and the risk of failure is all too real. In the concluding part of this book we'll look at a number of change issues and examine approaches that can help those who want to be champions of change. Chapter Ten provides a profile of do's and don'ts that can increase immensely the probability of pulling off a successful transformation. And Chapter Eleven provides a point-by-point outline of how to organize and sequence change.

Change doesn't just happen, and organizations don't change themselves. In the end, improving the world around us demands the intelligent application of principles of change and a committed heart that will accept nothing less than that the world becomes better. In the end, it all hinges on commitment.

Chapter Ten

Defeating the Limits of Change

Just the very thought of trying to change the organizations we work in is enough to make us despair. The experienced manager knows the difficulties, and they can be daunting. It's reminiscent of the Old Testament story of David and Goliath. The Philistine army had a big bully, Goliath, who each day would come out at high noon and bellow across the valley to the army of Israel that they should send a single soldier to fight him in a kind of World Wrestling Federation winner-take-all. Hearing this challenge, the quaking soldiers thought, "He's so big—I can't possibly kill him." But young David saw the problem differently: "He's so big—I can't miss!" It's pretty much like that in management. Once we see that any attack on the problem can't miss, everything becomes easier.

This chapter identifies some of the key issues that must be addressed for organizational upgrading to succeed. Indeed, research and experience show that the model of change is not as important to success as the process of how change is made, and whether there is enough energy to drive it, in determining eventual success or failure. We will look at the particularly difficult change terrain that is part of the health care system organization, understand the reasons that transformation efforts fail, and identify how to determine whether the organization has readiness for change. From this will emerge a number of axioms for success that the skilled change master can use in successfully steering departmental, organizational, or system-wide improvement.

System Building—A Questionable Track Record

In the current pursuit of answers for how to properly structure the health care industry, a widespread effort is being made to consolidate through acquisitions, mergers, and alliances, but these issues can take leaders away from the job of creating true high-performance organizations. Although the goals of the organizers are admirable, we need to ask, What are the outcomes? And what problems are commonly experienced in the new systems that are being formed? I don't want to be disheartening, just cautionary. Says Dwight Gertz, co-author of *Grow to Be Great*, "This rush for growth is going to create more losers than it does winners. Real growth is rare" (cited in Henkoff, 1996).

How Successful Are Acquisitions?

Buying or merging with another organization would seem to be the easiest way to get bigger faster. Will this be true for hospitals? It hasn't been in other industries. According to a McKinsey study, just 23 percent of acquisitions earned their cost of capital in deals made by 116 companies over an eleven-year period. An example is Quaker Oats, who paid $1.7 billion for Snapple, whose continued losses drained Quaker's earnings. Investors, who win only by understanding this common outcome, tend to shun stocks of acquiring organizations. As a result, a company's stock price tends to rise only 30 percent of the time when an acquisition is announced, because acquisitions prove to be financially successful only 23 percent of the time (Henkoff, 1996).

Often this failure is due to mismatching cultures, or lack of a clear picture of what each party will contribute or achieve by the merger. Unfortunately, consolidation is often driven by the desire for empire building more than sound business need. As Herb Kelleher, Southwest Airlines CEO, says, "To hell with market share. Grow with discipline to achieve profit" (Dunlap Godsey, 1996).

How Successful Are Alliances?

Another way of trying to achieve group strength is via alliances or coalitions. Although this is a popular option, what can we actually expect from it? Though it's still too early to tell how this approach will bear out in the hospital industry, experience elsewhere is not promising. One study of alliances from 1991 to 1996 surveyed over 2000 executives. When asked how well these partnerships met their strategic goals, they gave an average grade of B−. But when asked to rate the financial performance of those same alliances, the grade dropped to a C−. Typical of the problems reported was that the basic operations work necessary to get the partners going in the same direction wasn't done. Says Consultant Jordan Lewis, "The importance of having shared objectives seems obvious, but it's often overlooked. It's hard enough to get two departments of the same company to agree on the same thing" (Henkoff, 1996).

How Successful Are Systems?

While the jury is still out on whether health care systems will live up to their promise and are worth the trouble of organizing, there is no denying the logic in forming them.

- Greater purchasing power means lower costs. Shared services and overhead elements represent greater efficiencies.
- Common information and accounting systems allows less total overhead of these specialists, primarily through the productivity of computerization.
- Greater clout within regions sharpens competitive power, thus favoring the capture of market share.

However, whether systems are truly able to achieve these and other positive outcomes has yet to be proved. Although there is no question that some systems are or will be successful, the evidence suggests a rocky road and failure ahead for many.

- Systems seem to come and go as frequently as coaches for America's no-win sports teams. Remember Humana, HCA, and others who rode high for awhile, only to be subsumed in the next feeding frenzy? The purchasing of properties is easy, but running a system is hard. When one looks at the numbers and projected benefits on paper, forming such an enterprise seems like a wonderful idea, but operating a system is a lot harder than it looks.
- Many system executives were upgraded from single-facility leadership posts. Does their lack of experience in running a multi-unit business create problems? The report of many individual

hospitals is that system involvement has slowed decision making and is intrusive and often inappropriate to local market needs. This may prove to be simply a matter of time and experience, but system posts shouldn't be an on-the-job learning experience. Increasingly, systems will recognize the need for experienced executives from other industries who know how to manage large multiunit enterprises.

The continuing criminal allegations and ethical failures among systems executives reported in the press indicates less that people are venal or can fail, and more that systems encounter ill-defined law, fail to set up reporting systems that can spot problems before they reach crisis stage, and inadequately train leaders in how to avoid risks and traps. Perhaps the harshest judgment was that of one cynic, who noted that the development of many systems was for the eventual financial aggrandizement of the founders as they sell out in a frenzy of ever higher market prices, rather than for improved care of patients. It's not necessary to call people's motivations into question to observe that the operating environment is filled with many traps.

The Allina Health System, led by highly regarded CEO Gordon Sprenger, is often cited as a model for other systems. But at one point in time its integration problems were reported in the press this way (Scott, 1997): "Allina hasn't mastered the aligning part of alliances. Halfway into its third year of operation, the high-profile Minnesota health system is finding it hard to act like a unit. Part of the problem is Allina must be an integrated company, an independent provider network, and a separate health plan all at once to meet the demands of the Twin Cities market. More bothersome are its difficulties in forming the most vital link in the cost-control chain—physician cooperation in capping utilization."

The turbulence that even the best systems encounter often stems from external sources. In the Allina instance, vertically integrated systems were being pushed by state and federal authorities, which would have driven all payers and providers into such deals, but these reform efforts were ultimately abandoned. When external turbulence forces these realignments, it adds yet another distraction for leaders who need to focus on straightening out internal operations. It's hard to do system building under the best of circumstances, nearly impossible when outsiders keep pulling up the flowers to see whether the roots are growing.

If acquisitions, alliances, and systems have this kind of track record, why pursue them? Some organizations probably shouldn't. Yet there are compelling economic and organizational management reasons that consolidation should and will continue.

Are Health Systems Really Systems?

As we approach the question of how to standardize the health care industry, let's free ourselves from the illusion that systems are systems. This is a case where the marketing language has run ahead of an emerging management reality. Current health "systems" are actually collections, chains, or conglomerates. Their widely different procedures and methods represent little in the way of true management standardization. This is understandable, given that their members were for the most part acquired elements, rather than the offspring or clones of existing successful units.

"Integrated in Name Only" trumpeted the headline of one press report, faulting so-called health care networks. In a story primarily focused on inadequate information capability, the problems of nonsystemic "systems" were pilloried (Morrissey, 1998a):

> Like the storybook emperor who got caught in a fabric of fiction, health care delivery networks may be heading into the marketplace embarrassingly underdressed.
>
> These new conglomerations of care sites have a certain appeal —but only if they're clad in a stylish design called "integration."
>
> Executives who plunge ahead this year with business strategies based on integration should check first that they have done enough to weave information systems into their provider networks. If not, they won't have the substance behind the idea. . . .
>
> Even if payers buy into the integration promise, networks may be fooling themselves and undermining their bottom line if they accept risk for the well-being of patients only to find out they can't manage them without systems to follow their every move. Alas, they are "integrated delivery networks" in name only.

These conglomerates often have widely disparate cultures within them, leading to much internal conflict. Under the same corporate flag, different cultural entities war for dominance, as each partisan attempts to prevail in implanting his or her own limited background: "The way we did it at Edsel Memorial was better." Inevitably the old-boy, old-girl networks operate to make the new "system" a strange variant of the old from whence they came. Culture wars often underlie differences of leadership approach (participative, directive), operations execution (authority level, structure, training), or in program emphasis (home care, psychiatric). The yin-yang tug of war creates management casualties and considerable undesirable friction and wasted energy. The system, in truth, is more at risk from these self-defeating behaviors than from the threat of outside competitors.

The Need for System Debate

The German philosopher Georg Wilhelm Friedrich Hegel (1770–1831), a father of modern philosophy, sought to build a system of thought that encompassed all philosophy (see Taylor, 1979, and Strathern, 1997, for more on Hegel). Observing the seething forces of Europe in the early 1800s, he was particularly interested in the resolution of conflict and clash of ideas caused by major change, a topic of key interest to health care leaders today. He is most famous for the Hegelian dialectic, a force of reason that inevitably shapes the outcome of all conflict—a future predictor of results, if you will.

The dialectic goes like this: For every *thesis,* Hegel wrote, there is an opposite *antithesis.* These forces, organizations, people, and ideas will go through a period of conflict. In time the conflict produces a *synthesis,* not just a blend of ideas from both sides, but a higher order, and it is this synthesis that ultimately prevails and in turn becomes the thesis of yet another triad. Said more simply: "There's your way, there's my way, and there's the right way." A current example is communist China moving rapidly toward market capitalism to form a socialist capitalist state. So, too, must system managers move toward an elevated synthesis of their mixed inheritance, a higher plane of performance.

Management prescription. If Hegel is right, leaders should encourage open debate, *let no current positions dominate,* and force people into the underrepresented synthesis that represents the organization's true future.

A related idea of Hegel's was that the process of reason and logic was a surer perspective than the more limited empirical view. Translation: Bet on right thinking more than current experience. The management problem of standardization on best practices may be immense—it will be heated—but the outcome is certain: True health care excellence will emerge, but it will emerge a lot faster if leaders open up their departments, organizations, and systems to an open critique and rejection of the status quo.

Change Approaches Under Way: Which Will Succeed?

Regina Herzlinger, noted health strategist, has suggested in her book *Market Driven Health Care,* that the hospital industry has been pursing three "diets," three very different approaches in their efforts to adapt to the managed-care resource-scarce environment (Herzlinger, 1997):

1. Downsizing—the "just say no" diet. Many health care organizations have followed the downsizing road with the pain of multiple layoffs, chopping services, and accepting lower payment for services under managed care. Will this road lead to success? A quick summary of Herzlinger's argument is that it will not. Just as downsizing strategies failed in other industries, it will fail in health care. People can't starve their way to health, and organizations can't cost contain their way to excellence.

2. Upsizing—the "big is beautiful" diet. Creating larger organizations or systems through consolidation of local hospitals has tremendous allure. After all, isn't big more efficient? Isn't big better? Certainly it becomes possible to eliminate duplicated expenses, and some health care organization have been able to do this, particularly when looking at *horizontal integration* (where units are the same as in multiple surgicenters), which is difficult but doable. However, *vertical integration* (where units are dissimilar: hospital, home care, hospice, psychiatric) adds infinitely to the complexity of change that must be mastered. The experience in other industries shows that vertical integration usually results in failure, yet health care insists on revisiting this high-risk model.

3. Resizing—the "trade fat for muscle" diet. This is the hardest course to follow, for it requires rebuilding the operating system from the ground up. This is where Herzlinger makes her pitch for

the focused factory, a seamless and smooth system processing a limited number of diagnoses. Resizing, sometimes called *rightsizing,* has proven to be most successful in the rest of American industry. My own position is in this ballpark and is expressed as best practices standardization, focused on the necessarily wider range of cases that hospitals will have to serve for the near future. Common rightsizing tactics include outsourcing, spinning off business units not related to a defined market strategy like Operational Excellence, and getting rid of all extraneous projects and pursuits. This is the lean, mean, fighting machine that Herzlinger, and business experience, recommends.

Evidence is already accumulating that shows the fundamental errors of downsizing and upsizing diets. The headline in *Modern Healthcare* read, "Lesson Still Isn't Getting Through: Bigger Isn't Better" (1996): "Health care executives who are serious about ensuring the survival of their institutions know they must walk the walk—not simply talk the talk—of transformation. But amid the furious consolidation of nearly half the nation's hospitals into larger systems, some troubling sidesteps are evident. After the ink on the merger agreements dries, few institutions are making critical changes in service delivery and consolidating services to provide more effective care."

In a study by Deloitte & Touche, as reported in *Modern Healthcare* ("Lesson Still Isn't Getting Through," 1996), it was found that only 7 percent of respondents had cut or eliminated patient services when merging or joining larger organizations, thus losing the opportunity to combine services and achieve substantial efficiencies. It is interesting that the administrative side was where service consolidations had occurred (31 percent combined accounting and finance, 28 percent combined billing and collections)—perhaps because it was easier to do or politically more acceptable.

What emerges from these efforts are two essential understandings. First, in spite of whatever evidence may exist to the contrary, system building will continue apace in the hospital industry. Whether the battlefield is risky is immaterial, for the battle is joined. Some individual hospitals may decide to remain solo or stay in modest-sized systems where problems are more manageable, at least until some future time when some of the cloud over the battlefield has dissipated. But for most, the name of the game is "go system." The second understanding is the need to get under control the elements of change management that can reduce risk and maximize chances for success. Like surgeons dealing with high-risk surgery, we need to control as many factors as possible surrounding this operation if we are to increase chances for success.

Current experience suggests that hospital chains are putting their first standardization efforts into clinical protocols (where potentially huge gains can be made in both quality and cost), finance (get common financial reports for apples-to-apples measurement and consolidated reporting), information systems (a common basis for communications and a key foundational element for future standardization work), and purchasing (initially for substantial cost reduction, with future cost reductions coming from reducing the number of suppliers and supply variations). These are commonsense approaches that should produce substantial benefits.

However, this primarily economic and data-driven thrust is a flawed strategy that may prove inadequate for long-term results. The risk is that while standardizing these limited areas, the rest of the organization's functioning will remain widely variant. Unless clinical care protocols are really driven home, and unless support services procedures, human resource practices, and the culture itself become more standardized, the economic initiatives will provide only short-term balance-sheet improvement.

Systems in their current state of evolution face a number of other risks:

• Failure to build a business. Already we have seen the Illusory System, in which managers construct an organization rather than building a business. The assemblage of ill-fitting units makes it appear that there is a cohesive regional or national organization, rather than the uncomfortable grouping that is more often the case. Consolidation is insufficient and represents failure if there is no subsequent evolution into excellence.

• Too much autonomy. Some chains, in their discomfort over the control issue that is part of standardization, will fail to address it. The phrase "local control" seems to be the buzzword for this avoidance. In some instances, wise managements are allowing each operating unit to pursue its own course. Local control definitely has some value when a best practice approach has not been determined. However, once it is shown that one approach or another has proven itself, can top executives continue to allow lower performance results in approaches that have not produced? To some degree local control may be a luxury, particularly after better approaches are known, for it multiplies work and prolongs the time until all units are functioning at better levels. Local control assumes the specious argument that talent levels are the same in all units, that each has the ability and time to do the work, and that each can achieve better performance.

• Lack of speed. Another risk is going slow in moving toward standardization. Not only does slow approach delay the killer competitive advantages that standardization could represent, it fails to truly weigh the seriousness of the problem in the present. The forces at work suggest that the time window that allowed for non-standardization and lower standards has closed, and that the management challenge is to fix the performance gap now.

• Lack of decisiveness. A final risk area is that management, in dealing with uncertain times, will fail to move with certainty. This takes the form of settling for incremental organizational change, which seems more palatable and less disquieting, rather than going for the radical and rapid change to the New American Hospital model that is more appropriate for the times. Don't use bandages when surgery is called for.

Helping Organizational Change Efforts Succeed

An assessment of failed change programs in the hospital industry found certain recurring themes that led to failure. These often were the mirror reverse of elements found in successful interventions. The following common success factors tend to lead to desired outcomes:[1]

---

[1] This list combines the author's experience in over 700 health care organizations in assisting with widescale change efforts along with the findings of other organization development experts. Some of this material is taken from Otter (1995) and Schaffer and Thomson (1992).

1. View the change not as a program add-on, but as a new way of life. The risk lies in thinking that the organization is fundamentally OK and only needs tweaking. Much of the history of change efforts in the hospital world has been patch, patch, patch, which produces a crazy quilt. Often these patches last only as long as the careers of the executives who approved them. Change must be thought of as affecting the entire organization's processes. It is not just a piecemeal add-on. Adopt the mindset that we are entering a new way of thinking, acting, and speaking that will lead eventually to triumph.

2. Change leaders must approve content, not just concept. The theories are good behind TQM, reengineering, guest relations training, and the myriad of other programs that the industry has tried. Although the ideas were good, inserting them into daily practice proved infinitely more difficult than writing the check to pay for them. Promise thus outruns performance. Military strategists report that when a commander must choose between a superior plan that is likely to have average implementation versus one that is less good conceptually but likely to be superbly executed, choose the latter. Both ideas and execution must be correct to deliver best results.

3. Rely less on consultants. Externally derived curatives are seldom as effective as home-grown varieties. Help from consultants may be necessary but is seldom desirable, especially in terms of final program design and implementation. When one must be used, assume as much control and direct involvement of the organization's people as possible to get commitment and buy-in. No outsider, no matter how good, can understand the organization's needs and problems as well as the people who deal with them everyday. Make the organization their baby.

4. Focus on results, not process. If there has been one monumental error it has been the disproven notion that elevated "process, process, process" over simple results. Successful change masters know that too little in the way of results leads to initiative failure more than anything else. Nowhere was this more clearly seen than in the failure of TQM programs. Management is a results game. Get results any way you can as long as they're legal and ethical. The balancing counterargument is that when results are poor, look upstream at the lousy process that produces inadequate

output. The point is that results are primary, and process is secondary, not the other way around.

5. Establish a sense of urgency. People always seem to respond to emergencies and the big, important tasks. The problem in much of health care is that there are too many priorities and an endless clutter of requests. If the pursuit of best practices is to succeed it must be transformed to *best practices now.* Make people aware of the nasty realities of the market and competition. Don't keep the bad news from them. Identify and discuss crises and major opportunities. Set deadlines. Push, push, push.

6. Form a powerful guiding coalition. Any organization veteran knows that the person in charge of a project can spell life or death of an idea. When quality initiatives get sidelined to a small staff department, quality is going nowhere. Put together a group with the managerial muscle to do the task; get them really cooking as a team and then stand back. Commandos are taking the field.

7. Create and communicate the vision. Change efforts have a way of going off track because the terrain is always unfamiliar. The "vision thing" has value because it paints a broad picture of what the promised land is all about. It has both navigational and motivational value. But to succeed, vision has to be joined by tactics. Communication to the nth power becomes essential. Think of being in a dark forest, alone—keep shouting, "We're here. This is what's happening." Frequency of communication is also important (how about daily "Change Grams"?), as is face-to-face, and "just the facts" reporting.

8. Empower others to act on the vision. This translates to a number of specific actions that remove the organization's depowering influences. Get rid of obstacles to change ("no time, untrained, never been done before, policies don't permit"). These things undermine the vision and are akin to shooting yourself in the foot. The damn system works at every turn to kill the future you're trying to create. Get an attitude about cutting through the crap and red tape. Insist on nontraditional ideas and actions. Create an environment of safety that tolerates mistakes.

9. Plan for and create short-term wins. If I ask my kids, "Would you like $1 today or $10 a year from today?" they invariably take the buck. I assume that's because of their high intelligence rather than an unwillingness to trust me for that long. People want re-

inforcement for their behavior, and they want it now. If you were dating, would you want feedback the night of the first date, perhaps a goodnight kiss, or would you rather have a full performance review in a year? Because success breeds success, plan for some highly visible wins and improvements, then celebrate those wins. It keeps the worker bees flying, and gives credence to the notion that this just might be the right course.

10. Consolidate improvements, produce more change. Ultimately, the program must produce a prodigious amount of change. As the program gains initial credibility, let it also gain in number of participants and volume of change. As the train rolls down the track, remove those few people who don't fit the vision and bring on board those who do, and reinvigorate the process with new projects, themes, and change agents.

An Example of Change Mastery

During the Gulf War, operations were divided into two elements, Desert Shield and Desert Storm. Desert Shield was the approximately three month build-up of materials and manpower. Getting everybody and everything in place before launching the attack meant that there would be fewer shortages, screw ups, and failed missions. General Gus Pagonis was responsible for this portion of the war effort. His remarkable success made Desert Storm possible, and his leadership provided a number of valuable insights on how to get at change management problems (Pagonis, 1992):

- [At regular] "skull sessions," [I would invite] a large group of people from many functional areas into one room and lead them through a discussion of how they would handle a range of hypothetical-but-plausible challenges. The goal . . . is to do our Monday-morning quarterbacking on Saturday night.
- [The] theater was so large that I couldn't be in enough places often enough. Recognizing that fact, I deputized a group of soldiers—dubbed the "Ghostbusters"—as my proxies. They went into the desert as my official eyes and ears, making sure everything was running smoothly, giving and gaining a clearer sense of the theater's overall organization.
- Formal methods of information transfer are very important, but I find that you don't get a complete view of what's actually

happening in an organization unless you also open regular informal communication channels. For straight talk, nothing compares with the comments I pick up during my daily basketball game with the troops.

A key to success is that planning the standardization effort needs to be very operational in nature, and divided between a preparation wave and the actual rollout of the implementation. Nothing happens because of a plan. Don't lose the opportunity by failing the test of mastering the nitty-gritty.[2]

Creating the System Organization

Let's begin by looking at where system building has been at least moderately successful. These suggestions make things easier for leaders trying to elevate performance across a multi-unit system:

- Start small. Working with a smaller group of organizations rather than a large group reduces complexity. Larger systems should consider standardization within a region, or by type of facility, rather than trying to do all at the same time.
- Try horizontal integration first. Horizontal integration (example: hospital to hospital) and standardization has far more likelihood of success than vertical integration (hospital with extended care and home care). If the situation allows, perhaps attacking horizontal integration first will provide a stable platform of success to help win support when the vertical integration efforts begin. Following the same strategy, perhaps all home care operations in the system can be standardized before rotating the next organizational element.
- Provide common languages and tools. Health care is a tower of Babel, a polyglot of professional tongues and technospeak. Commonality can be increased via training on values, the new

---

[2]The reader is directed to the author's companion book, *Creating the New American Hospital, a Time for Greatness,* for a fuller description on change implementation techniques and solutions in leading wide-scale organizational change. The focus of the book is how to renew a single-facility organization, though much of its findings are also applicable to a multi-unit system.

culture, and problem-solving approaches that all will use, such as continuous improvement tools or Do It Groups. Push for elements of a common worldview. Tie these elements together with the infrastructure backbone of computerization and ready information flow.

- Add the element of common skills training. One hospital found they were following three different techniques for doing blood draws. Reduction of process variations leads to greater flexibility in staffing and increased quality. It provides the basis for cross training between departments and between job descriptions.

System building has been less successful where it follows the old management approaches of a long string of mandates and compulsory programs. That is not to say that there shouldn't be a clear structure and proper direction and somebody putting some urgency into the situation. The risk of a noninvolved, powered-down set of field organizations is that the good people will leave, the organization won't learn to think for itself, and the loss of intellectual capital will severely damage the business. So there is a necessary blending between how participative and patient leaders can be, and how directive they must be.

Assessing an Organization's Readiness for Change

An organization's need for change and its readiness for change are two entirely separate issues. The business may be in trouble in terms of quality, cost, and Customer and human outcomes, but there may not be a corresponding readiness of that organization to change. Some executives have naively assumed that all that would be required would be to announce the program of the month, see the heads bobbing up and down at management meetings, and watch perfection unfurl within the organization.

Change becomes more difficult to pull off if the organization's goals are being met. Organizations that are in trouble, and know it, have a far greater probability of success in making change precisely because everybody understands that changes must be made. Hence the saying, "Things will have to get worse before they get better." Still, there has to be enough to work with; that is, the business must still be viable. There has to be some market share, there has to be at least borrowing capability if funds are exhausted, and there has to be a small cadre of management talent to lead the change, the kind of people you'd want with you in a foxhole.

Right now morale may be a little down. If you don't sense that people are positive or excited, yet they're good folks, some cheerleading might help. More important, the magic ingredient of good leadership could challenge and uplift them. Is it possible to spend some time to get people talking and excited about change? What articles could be sent around showing success stories? What meetings or parties could be held? If you want to go forward and believe that the values and substance of your group can rekindle the fire, you may be ready for change.

And what about the political climate? How are board relations, and interaction with physicians? Will differences of opinion and debate be within normal range or not? If you're part of a system, will the system provide enough autonomy, or will there be critics on the sideline? One wise CEO waited an entire year to make change so that he could bring his board members on board! When major change commences, not every report from the front that reaches the ear will be positive. Problems will happen, mistakes will be made, and you don't want to have the political ground go cold just short of bringing home the trophy. If you want to go forward and understand how you will bring along the other power players, you may be ready for change.

Are organization executives ready to deal with outliers and Stalinists, those who stonewall against the change, outright resist it, or silently sabotage it? Only the naive think we're all going forward as a team with great enthusiasm and happiness as we contemplate the Promised Land. Moses could have gotten his people there in a week's walk if they'd been a team. It's been said he had to wander around in the desert for forty years to let the resisters and drags die off. Are we ready to lose a few managers if they don't want to go on the journey to twenty-first century health care? If you want to go forward, in spite of having to face up to some tough personnel decisions, you may be ready for change.

As a practical matter, there is never an ideal time to make change because every organization is always busy, always has too much on its plate. Ask the question of your management team: Is this an acceptable time to make change? Can we control the flow of other work and sustain the change initiative as a priority? Would we be better off to put off the change? Starting is easy, finishing is tough. That's why they don't hand out the prize until you cross the finish line. Is it doable given the work load? Can we afford to wait? If you want to go forward, now, in spite of the work, you may be ready for change.

A Change Readiness Checklist

Below are a number of other key elements that indicate readiness for change. To be sure that the organization is in a state of readiness, use the following checklist. Rate your organization on each item by checking off the areas you have covered. Circle items that need considerable work. This can be done by a group of managers to get a more complete picture.

Experience shows that the cluster of responses, their pattern, seems to be most descriptive and helpful. A profile with many of the elements won't guarantee success of the change initiative, but it can give a good indication that the effort is not premature or ill-timed, and that there are enough of the components present that favor a good outcome. Likewise, if lots of the elements are weak or missing, it doesn't mean that change can't be pulled off, just that it will be more difficult and the plan and its execution need to be well designed.[3]

• *Does the business need to change?* Do improvement needs exist? They do if the organization is in trouble, or knows it needs to improve in one or more of its key success factors of cost, Customer satisfaction, and quality, or has internal staff morale problems. Deficiencies in these areas tend to create a burning platform where people will work with you for change.

• *Is there a powerful change sponsor?* Is the sponsor of change a person with enough power in the organization to pull it off? This

---

[3] Elements in the list are taken from the author's "Organization Performance and Readiness Assessment," an organization diagnostic tool, supplemented with some ideas from "Rate Your Readiness to Change," *Fortune*, February 7, 1994.

is usually the CEO or COO. He or she has the vision and will play the role of chief cheerleader and will deal with resistance when it occurs. Sponsors at lower levels have less chance of success. Are the power-people willing to sacrifice perks or power for the good of the group? Does the magnitude of change contemplated fit with the power of the person driving it?

• *Does senior management want change?* Do they want a different future and have they articulated what it should look like? Do they have the ability to mobilize all of the relevant parties? If they think only small or program change is needed, rather than major systemic change, the likely outcome is no change at all.

• *Can a high degree of program leadership be mobilized?* These are the people who oversee things, set the goals, work until midnight. Change is likely to succeed when high-level leaders are involved and there is enough participation and cooperation to encompass the area(s) of the organization being changed, enough direct responsibility and freedom to carry out tasks, and clear business goals to achieve. As above, does the magnitude of change contemplated fit with the power of the person driving it?

• *Is there a sense of urgency and motivation?* This has to start from senior management and be sold to the rest of the organization. Add points if there is a culture that already emphasizes continuous improvement. Deduct points if people have been in their jobs for more than ten years or there is a conservative culture that discourages taking risks.

• *Are measures and rewards tied to goals?* Do measures exist that are related to specific improvement targets (cycle time reduction, cost improvement percentages) or BHAG objectives (95th percentile on national standards of Customer satisfaction)? Are rewards tied to achievement? If they are not present, can they be added quickly?

• *Will the change effort fit?* Will it fit in with other program initiatives that already have organizational momentum? Will it fit with the existing culture and philosophy of the organization? Does it dovetail with new acquisitions or other organizational entities that may be tangentially involved? Change will be easier if the new puzzle piece fits with the others already on the board.

• *Will process changes be welcome?* Organizational change, because it is major, almost invariably means redesigning procedures and processes, often across departmental lines. If empire builders are turf sensitive, that will slow things down. Is there good problem solving now in the team, or will this be a resistance area?

- *Is the organization outward referencing?* Are the people affected by the change sufficiently professional that they reference what competitors and other benchmarks are doing to get objective comparisons? Or are they primarily internal referencing, justifying the "way we do it here," and providing anecdotal stories of local success rather than numbers that prove their point?

- *Is the political climate positive?* Are other players and stakeholders outside the change group going to be sufficiently supportive to allow change to happen? Is there enough agreement between internal and external parties so that political crosswinds won't interfere?

- *How good is the management team?* Are they brighter than the average bear, or, when looking into their eyes do you have to ask, "Is anybody home"? Is there a history of sustained management development, or are they simply promoted from the ranks and handled a title with no preparation? It's hard to win with a team of losers. It's hard to lose with winners. Does this area need a lot of work?

- *Is Customer focus weak or strong?* Is the value of Customer service alive and well, or are people just going through the motions? Do people know who their Customers are, know their needs, and have direct contact with them? If there's a lot of Customer focus it's relatively easy to get people agreeing to change to serve them better.

- *Does the reward system reinforce risk taking and innovation?* People are more willing to look for new solutions when there is positive recognition for it. Team-based, merit-based, and incentive compensation plans are better than step increases and cost-of-living adjustments, for the latter reward continuity and the status quo. Are there other nonfinancial rewards: Is the organization used to saying "thanks" a lot and in fun ways? Test: Are managers supported when they fail in positive efforts?

- *Is the organizational structure rigid or flexible?* No change in the organizational structure in the last five years is a negative, as are too many reorganizations. The best situation is one in which changes have been infrequent and well thought out.

- *How effective is internal communication?* Is it the same old boring newsletter, or are organizational channels up, down, and sideways wide open? Is it one-way or two-way? Test: Have we established a sense of communion and community? When change hits, confusion reigns. Communication is the antidote.
- *Is the organization hierarchy "lean and mean?"* The fewer levels of hierarchy and employee grade levels, the more likely an effort to change will succeed. Lots of layers of middle management and staff slow decision making can also create large numbers of people with the power to block change.
- *What's the change track record?* If the organization is worn out with change, if there seems to be an ever-changing list of "programs of the month," that indicates that the past change history has been unsuccessful or left a residue of resentment. Future change will also be unsuccessful unless some new way to approach it is found. A successful change history, on the other hand, tends to show people how to succeed, and forms bands and bonds that are helpful with new challenges.
- *Is the army up for the fight?* Mistrust, low team spirit, few volunteers are a bad sign. If people like each other, if trust between departments and between staff and management is present, change is a lot easier. Your army isn't going to beat anybody else if it's beating up on itself. A sample test: Is physician verbal abuse of staff allowed?
- *How innovative is the organization?* If there's a lot of red tape, multiple signatures required for approval, and a big emphasis on policy and procedures, people are discouraged from just getting together to get the job done. The best case is when there is good turn-around time, encouragement of lots of ideas and experimentation, and cooperative work between departments instead of divisional warfare.
- *Are decisions made rightly?* They are if they're made quickly, are on the right issues, and take into account the relevant facts and viewpoints. If they take forever, are made by the remote "them," with a lot of conflict during the discussions and blaming after decisions are announced, it's a liability. Change will require lots of decisions and a short time table.

Even if a lot of these areas aren't right, change is still possible. Some things can be fixed. People can be persuaded. Tradeoffs can be made. Look within. How fed up with what's going on are you? How badly do you want to make a difference? With or without you, everything around you will be changed in time.

Conclusion

In this chapter we've looked at the difficulties that health care organizations are having in forming mergers, alliances, and systems and the problems these difficulties create for installing best practices. Beyond questions of organizational structure, the real heart of the change problem comes when the standardization of procedures and improvement of culture are attempted. These difficulties are manageable and are begun by assessing readiness for change, and then using the positive prescriptions that favor successful change implementation. In the concluding chapter we will look at a sequential, step-by-step procedure to actually change the organization into an example of Operational Excellence.

Work-Out Session

1. Individually or as a group, list characteristics that represent positive forces or characteristics in your change situation— these are driving forces.
2. Now list the negative forces or elements in your situation— these are restraining forces.
3. Next, list ways in which you could reinforce or add to the driving forces.
4. Finally, list what could be done to remove or reduce the restraining forces.
5. Remember, managing the tough situations is why they gave you the title. What does your own inventory of self say you want to do with this situation?

Chapter Eleven

Transforming Health Care Organizations

In this book I have argued that the ultimate transformation of American health care rests on an across-the-board approach that sets and implements dramatically higher standards and standardizes all activity around best practices. I have shown the positive fit between standardization and the Operational Excellence strategy. Organizations that move in this direction stand a better chance of satisfying market requirements.

In this chapter we'll examine how to proceed with transforming our organizations to this higher ground. It's been said, however, that the problem with life is that it doesn't follow the policy manual. Making real change is a lot harder than it looks. Many leaders can relate to George Carlin, who said, "I put money in a change machine. Nothing changed!" Leaders need a path to follow in transformation work, step-by-step suggestions that will make possible moving from where the organization is now to where they want to take it. It is this road map to becoming a new American health care organization that becomes the last vital element leading to success.

A Step-by-Step Approach to Standardization

Experience has shown that organizational renaissance around the concept of standardizing best practices needs several elements to succeed. First, it needs a sound philosophical and conceptual basis that can answer fundamental business questions: What Customer need are we trying to serve? What market position will that require? What kind of organization can get us there? Second, there must be an aggressive approach to implementation, one that achieves rapid and massive change without falling victim to the traps that have foiled other change initiatives. This is an even more acute risk in systems that are being built, often cobbled, together. Third, all of this change effort must eventually produce not just activity, but action; not just "busy-ness," but business results.

Figure 11.1 illustrates how this might be undertaken. Consider this a generic outline, a beginning draft that can be detailed and tailored to the unique needs of each organization. Pictured are the fundamental elements that can serve as headlines for the total picture. The diagram works well for standardization within a single organization or a multi-unit system. It breaks the change down into three primary phases. The first is deciding course, which is the prechange work of organizing and reaching agreement as to philosophical fit and project objectives. The second phase is implementing change, in which change agents and change strategies are decided, standards and best practices are identified, and the work rolls out. The final phase is to direct change toward the work targets of Operational Excellence, the implementation of tactical plans for high satisfaction, high quality, low cost, and best people.

Deciding the Course

The first step is to look before leaping. Remember the old military saying, the one George Custer should have memorized: "The way in is easy, the way out is hard." This is a daunting amount of work. Proceed deliberately, not slowly, to understand all the dimensions of the project. Don't be afraid of the mountain, but look, and think, before you leap.

Change Czar

Usually organizations put an executive in charge of the overall effort (this job cannot be assigned to a staff department), often the CEO in an individual organization, but the task can be delegated to one of the more powerful and better VPs. It must be made clear to all that the project not only has the complete support of the chief executive, but that she will take an activist role, particularly

Figure 11.1. An Approach to Standardization.

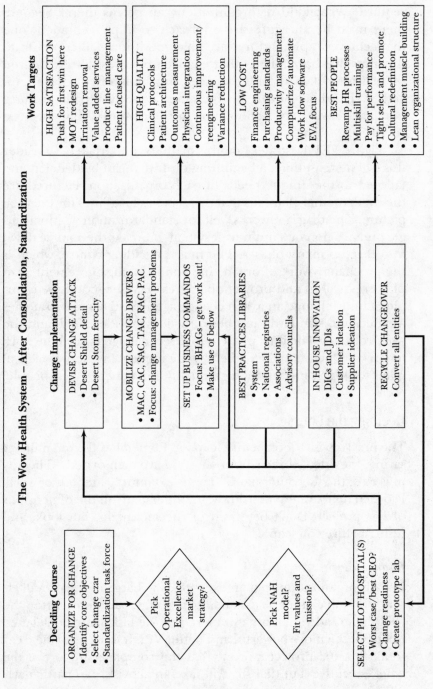

The Wow Health System – After Consolidation, Standardization

in explaining the program to staff. Management of the effort can be delegated; leadership of the people cannot.

The project leader usually begins by gathering people and information. The box in Figure 11.1 labeled "mobilize change drivers" often fits at this point in a single hospital but would usually be deferred until later in a system. No matter, what counts at this point is getting a cluster of people together, either as a task force or on an ad hoc basis, to do some brainstorming, blue-skying, and bull-throwing. The group needs to resolve some basic issues: Is this something we really need and want to do? Is it doable given the press of other work? Is the timing right? Do we have the change readiness in the organization? Can we do this on our own or will we need an outside guru? What do we hope the benefits will be? What costs will we have to pay? After some initial conferencing, people will often run for data to support their points of view. At this point there should be a full planning conference to reach a go/no-go decision that standardization is an appropriate approach for the organization.

Key Strategy Decisions

Once the decision to go ahead is firm and the change czar and her group begin to feel like they have their feet under them, two primary decisions need to be made, and those decisions need to be reality tested:

What does the market strategy need to be? As explained in Chapter Two, my view is that this should be an Operational Excellence (low-cost) strategy. What changes and improvements on this thinking would the group want to offer? Can these be made while still avoiding the trap of trying to be everything to everybody? The point of reviewing this question now is that one doesn't want to reengineer the organization in a way that is at variance to the needed market strategy: The organization is an extension of the strategy, not the other way around.

What type of organization should we build? The organizational prototype most likely to deliver needed business results is the New American Hospital, which is briefly described in Chapter Six (see Sherman, 1993, for a fuller discussion). Does the change task force agree with this assessment? What other options do we want to explore? If the objective is to get a man on the moon, don't build a train as the vehicle.

One way to assess whether the organization model you want to create and the strategy you want to pursue are appropriate is to review the organization's values and cultural history. These core values serve as an excellent *test for fit*. A problem for newly minted systems is that they are often a hodgepodge of histories, and along with building the new system they have to forge a new culture. Without it, every decision becomes a minor war, a swamp of resistance. What do we stand for? Does the program of change we're thinking about entering fit with what we are, and what we are trying to become?

Select the Pilot

At this point, the change team will want to select a pilot hospital, if part of a system, or check to make sure elements of change readiness are present if dealing with a single organization. Under no circumstances should you try to achieve organizational renewal across the entire system at once. (There can be some exceptions for that rule when the system is small.) The pilot hospital represents the opportunity to get the bugs out of your design, and to learn from errors in content, sequence, and methods of delivery. This is particularly important when the changeover is going to be driven without expert assistance.

Criteria for selecting the pilot organization include the following:

• Degree of current success. Change is often easier to pull off in organizations struggling to survive. In the turnaround of the Chrysler Corporation there was a remarkable readiness to change; everyone knew the organization was on the verge of filing Chapter 11. Jobs were on the line, and everyone was ready to cooperate. However, in the successful organization, people don't see the need for change; they keep up a continuous patter of how good they think they are, thus exhibiting the pride that goes before a fall. If there is a choice that can be made, picking the sicker organization might be the best decision.

• Strength of leadership. Does the CEO have the horsepower, energy, and drive to lead a sustained charge? Does she have the interpersonal skills to handle the communication load that will be so important? Does he have the vision to see the possibilities of a new day, and the commitment to get there in spite of all obstacles?

What about the middle managers? Are they bright enough? Are they fed up sufficiently with the status quo?

• Presence of Big D. Dissatisfaction energy (Big D) drives organizational change more than the positive desire to make things better. Both energy sources are important, but it is the deeply felt anger, fear, or remembrance of pain or death of a loved one that has been found to fuel resolve most forcefully for change. Upset physicians, lawsuits, fear of loss of employment are sources of energy—energy needed to make change. The skilled change leader doesn't fear this negative energy but releases it toward positive ends. Lots of Big D is predictive of success.

If Big D is lacking, two possible avenues around the problem are possible. First, create dissatisfaction by focusing on the negatives, which are always present even in the best organizations. Amplify them, communicate them, target them. Doylestown Hospital in Doylestown, Pennsylvania, awards the "Vernon," a beat-up plastic pink flamingo yard ornament, to the form, procedure, or process that is felt to be in need of fixing. The Vernon is awarded monthly in good fun to the department manager, but no manager wants to receive this prize two months in a row.

Another way to stir up Big D is to have an "on-fire" executive light a candle under those who still think all is well in Happy Valley. Lawrence Bossidy, CEO of Allied Signal and one of America's best change executives, says, "You learn early in the change business that you've got to break some legs." This kind of talk may be hard for high-consideration, low-structure managers to hear, but being completely, even abruptly, honest about where things stand is essential. An organizational awareness that there is zero tolerance for certain behaviors and attitudes is important. Excellence is not always comfortable, nor should it be.

The pilot hospital becomes a learning lab, a place where imperfections teach us what to do next. At this stage it is better to underpromise and overdeliver. What you're trying to achieve is an example that can be shown to the rest of the system. On more than one occasion Wal-Mart has chosen its poorest performing store, and assigned to it a group of usually younger, up-and-coming managers with the order to turn it into the best-performing unit in the chain. What an opportunity. Later, when other managers say, "How did they get such great numbers?" they are told, "Go to

Dubuque." The pilot can become an internal benchmark—the pattern to follow.

Implementing the Renewal Plan

The second and major phase of the work is in implementing the total wave of change and implementing best practices throughout the house.

Create a Change Strategy and Work Plan

There is a high mortality rate for change programs in American hospitals. Although they are in the midst of a sea change, a true revolution in organizational management approach, these hospitals come to the battlefield with soldiers who are worn out from past failed efforts at changing the status quo. Analyses of failed programs reveals two central truths:

1. Use a reasonably good change model. Most change models, the defined content of the changes to be made, have reasonably acceptable content. They usually contain good ideas needed by the business. Whether they are for guest relations, continuous improvement, or reengineering, the logic and business potential are usually positive. Although these models for change are good, they will not succeed by themselves. One comes to the conclusion that change models are a dime a dozen. Every new management text has them (including this one), and every consultant and seminar offers them. A good model and fifty cents buys a cup of coffee. You've got to have one, so find the best one you can, and make it appropriate to your organization.

2. Implementation must be superior. Experience has shown that sometimes a less than best plan achieves far better results than other models that are judged superior. What accounts for the difference is that the implementation was superior. Since finding models is relatively the easier problem, spend most of the effort in thinking through the implementation challenges.

Where the real focus of work has to be is in thinking through how the change will be made. This is always important, but absolutely crucial when dealing with the magnitude of change that organization-wide change calls for. Hope that this will be a friendly and positive process, but make preparations as though you are going to war. This is difficult and detailed work, so make preparations thoroughly and thoughtfully. There are several elements that should be considered:

1. Get totally organized. We're talking about all the project management tools, Gantt charts, flow charts, calendars, resource budgeting, and all the stuff that has to be done to keep track of what's to be done, who's doing it, when and where it's happening, and who is accountable.
2. Identify what the key political and special interest concerns are going to be. Identify individuals or constituencies who may resist; do the same in identifying proponents. What are their issues?
3. Look at whether there should be special efforts made to align people in terms of the political world that exists in your shop.
4. Examine the ongoing work agenda. Can the change be calendared into a time window that is favorable given the press of other work?
5. Deal with the logistics questions: meeting rooms, communication channels, secretarial support, duplication. Set up a command headquarters. One hospital named theirs the Genesis Room.

Mobilize Change Drivers

In a single hospital, the original task force usually evolves into the coordinating groups that run the changeover. In a system, the task force may take this approach or may choose to delegate the implementation. We have found it useful to organize around various change functions with the following groups:

MAC—Management Action Council

This group of six to nine becomes the chief change contractor. The strongest middle managers often compose the group; there may be one executive member who serves as liaison. The MAC may report directly to the change czar if she is not on the MAC, or directly to the CEO if there is no one person to whom the project has been entrusted. However structured, the MAC is wired to the executive throne.

The group makes assignments of tasks, runs the Gantt charts, keeps track of overall progress, handles political interface, manages problems that crop up, and acts with wide authority. In terms of their freedom and range of action they might be likened to an unofficial vice president of change.

TAC—Training Action Council

A single hospital will need sixteen to twenty trainers to handle the dissemination of the many new skills needed in the organization to create empowerment at working levels. Course modules to define organization vision and values, skills training in small group problem solving, continuous improvement tools, managing departmental priorities and budgets, and numerous other elements are delivered by this group. The TAC chair is a member of the MAC, as are the chairs for the other groups detailed below.

The goal for training in the first year is forty hours of instruction, a benchmark obtained from excellent companies. Training is secondarily concerned about learning; it is primarily focused on getting people ready, willing, and able to carry out widescale change. Training is the springboard to setting up hundreds of problem-solving groups. A rule of thumb is that a hospital will run in the first year of changeover a number of groups equal to the number of full-time Associates.

SAC—Socialization Action Council

A hospital has poorly knit social patterns. Either people don't know each other (sometimes true of people working different shifts in the same unit) or, worse, have interdepartmental animosity. Four to five people known for their social and party skills are given the mission to "friendly up" the management team who are undergoing extensive management development. The goal is to create a leadership team in the hospital that knows each other, trusts each other, and will work hard together. To a large degree this means that people have to learn to play together first. Cheering contests, karaoke, calisthenics, riverboat trips, Pictionary, extemporaneous toasting, and costume parties are the order of the day. Later, this effort will spread to Associates as well. Although this may seem foolish to the old Neanderthals, we're forced to have fun, for it is another benchmark practice widely associated with excellence in performance. If you can't have fun, you can't make excellence.

RAC—Recognition Action Council

Many new behaviors are involved in converting and modernizing the old hospital. Change means ambiguity and some anxiety. People must be systematically reinforced and rewarded for mastering change and demonstrating the new behaviors. Totally unlike the old hospital, one is recognized for every idea submitted, every skill mastered, every step toward the goal. It's just like scouts —learn, do, and get a patch. Most rewards are no-cost or low-cost items (movie tickets, certificates, free lunch ticket), though a few big-ticket items are thrown in, just to keep it interesting (a trip to the Poconos). The idea is simply to pay attention to people and their successes, and by doing so encourage them to keep trying.

CAC—Communication Action Council

This small group struggles to keep people updated on the swirling vortex of change that is engulfing them. "Change Grams" on the cafeteria table daily, paycheck stuffers, in-house TV, town criers, e-mail, and departmental credible communicators and action reporters are all used to get the word out quickly. Gone are the dreary monthly newsletters with their carefully couched and multiply reviewed paragraphs. The organization begins to operate in real time. It's the What's Happenin' Now Hospital.

PAC—Physician Action Council

As Customer, Associate, and work leader, the physician's tri-part role requires identifying their needs and starting to shape the hospital in ways that serve their interests proactively, thus putting an end to reactive greasing of squeaky wheels. Young activist and older influential physicians help meld professional and organizational interests together. The fear that "physicians won't like it" turns out to be myth. Experience has shown that the reactions from physicians has been beneficial in every case, primarily because they can see demonstrated results and that others are going in the same direction. However, at the outset, before results are seen, it is likely that skepticism may be heard.

All of these groups are given the primary mission to organize and support the overall change effort. Although they are driving the change process, the actual specific work changes are driven by business commando teams. Think of the change-driver teams as creating the support climate for change, while the commando teams focus primarily on getting the change list accomplished.

Set Up Business Commando Teams

The organization's strategy is wedded to the standardization effort by setting up four commando teams to identify and then produce the needed work required to accomplish business purposes. The teams often choose names to define their mission:

High satisfaction—"Customer Commandos"

High quality—"Quality Questers"

Low cost—"Efficiency Special Forces"

Best people—"Associate Advocates"

These groups attempt to achieve established stretch goals (BHAGs) for their respective strategy element by attacking the many tasks that need doing: newer procedures, fewer policies, better tools, information loops and communication scoops, forms that help, fewer required signatures, new relationships, and an end to boundaries. What a lot of fun this is, especially when the numbers begin to change and show movement toward the goal. Liftoff!

Best Practices Libraries

Rather than starting from scratch, it's always more time efficient to use existing ideas, procedures, and practices that others have found to work. Your own creativity can then be added to the mix, building on what others have already done. Chapter Nine explained the idea of best practices. Sources of these ideas can be found from professional associations, consultants, universities, and the general management and technical literature. If the hospital is part of a system, it makes sense to establish a library to house these structural components of intellectual capital. Gathered together, these resources provide one-stop shopping to hospitals in that system. In a single hospital, the task remains one of pulling the requisite pieces together.

In-House Innovation

Under the leadership of the commando teams, hundreds of Do It Groups (DIGs, problems requiring a group) and Just Do Its (JDIs, problems assigned to individuals) are launched. The commandos can initiate and direct many of these by virtue of following the long list of recommendations for change worked out in our planned series, *Strategies for Health Care Excellence* (see Preface). But the majority of DIGs and JDIs come from the active imagination of Associates and unit leaders. The exciting phenomenon, an organization magic, is that once the call goes out for change and once people are trained and empowered to make that change, people find all kinds of things that need to be fixed, thus sparking a kind of spontaneous generation of solutions.

In the first year, nearly all change results from the work of Associates, leaders, involved physicians, and volunteers—members all of the hospital family. There is so much to do that there really isn't much time to involve any others. In the second and third years of organizational development, it is more feasible to involve Customers and patient families more widely, not just in focus groups but on problem-solving teams. Vendors conferences and the pursuit of the virtual corporation, in which one can't tell where the hospital ends and suppliers and Customers begin, becomes the new horizon for release of ideation.

Recycle Changeover

For the single hospital, this is the end of the conversion journey. In a system, once the pilot(s) is up and running, the process rolls through the rest of the system. This can be done in a kind of geometric progression, assuming training and support systems can handle it. Otherwise there will need to be a rotational strategy whereby those with experience help field units make the journey. Often the question of how fast one can push the standardized model through the system depends more on political acceptance than on the job of how to manage the change itself. How long can you wait for the benefits of standardization?

Pick Your Targets

What types of standardization work might go on in each of the four strategy areas? It's important to keep the overall organization transformation focused on business results. And the work items must all share the orientation that we are striving to implement proven best practices to achieve higher standards. Each implemented idea that shares that philosophy and managerial view, and that has been screened for fit with the organization's values, brings us a step closer.

The following lists are representative of the tasks, projects, and programs with which each BHAG council might flesh out as its overall "To Do" list for the year (see Tables 11.1 to 11.4). Our experience is that the work list that evolves in each team usually encompasses several hundred work items, some big, some small, all of which are needed. Because sources of ideas include internal ideation from everyone, along with best practices libraries externally, there's usually no shortage of things that need doing. Each BHAG council therefore needs to set some priorities without repressing what needs to be a torrent of change. As a general guideline, have an expectation that each tactical plan that results will include several hundred items for implementation within the following twelve months. Although this number may be staggering to some, experience has demonstrated that organizations tend initially to underestimate the amount of work that needs doing. Dabbling or surface skimming won't force deep enough or wide enough change to affect the organization, as revealed by later measurement.

The reader can also obtain a far more detailed listing of suggested changes from our best practices library, along with guidelines on how to implement them, in a series of implementation guides written as companion volumes to the present work on each of the BHAG areas (visit our website at managementhouse.com).

The next task is one of converting identified needs into a tactical plan by setting priorities, establishing the calendar, making assignments, and determining approach. This task converts the beginning lengthy list of hopes, projects, wishes, and problems into something real in terms of "what are we going to do next and who's going to do it?" Management's job is to convert information

Table 11.1. High Customer Satisfaction.

Tactical Plan Elements

Break down BHAG into quarterly work agendas

Set standards and guarantees

Identify and remove irritations

Identify and add value items

Pick moments of truth priorities

Target first and last impressions particularly

Physician account management and priorities

Patient focused care or other customer model

Facilities redesign for customer convenience

Street signage on internal halls

Intensify and simplify communications

Guest relations training

Patient for a day (staff training)

Adopt-a-patient program (each patient visited)

Healing environment retrofit

Work/job redesign for continuity of care

Service line management—organize around the Customer

Identify business coalition needs

Payer account management and priorities

Items affecting "likelihood to recommend"

Identify subset needs by age, sex, payer, etc.

Establish monthly and weekly customer metrics (Set specific subgoals to reach by date: e.g., % excellent, likely to recommend scores)

into action, and tactical plans help to accomplish that (a example format is found in Table 11.5).

The tactical plan is organized by quarter so that higher priority items come earlier in the year. Other criteria that affect placement or sequence of the tasks to be done during the year are items that will generate immediate positive press for the change program, Customer satisfaction priorities, workload issues, availability

Table 11.2. High-Quality Outcomes.

Tactical Plan Elements

Break down BHAG into quarterly work agendas

Departmental best practices program

Cycle time reduction program

Physician integration into quality initiatives

Evaluate/increase physician continuing ed

"Second opinion" computerized diagnostics

Computerization for seamless information

Standardize clinical protocols

Standardize supplies, reduce supplier number (Users make final decision, not purchasing)

Smooth patient transfers
  Physician to physician
  Physician to hospital
  Department to department

Rapid-fire continuous improvement

Cleanliness standards? (gum/cigarettes at front door?)

Dress standards? (jeans, clothing stains?)

Evaluate organization responses to errors

Standardize patient areas administrative layout

Standardize patient management layout

Exploit automation opportunities

Act on high variance, high-risk processes

Start-to-finish process improvement by service

Consider additive process improvement (breakthrough benchmarking in critical areas)

Patient architecture changes

Monthly and weekly outcomes metrics (Set specific subgoals to reach by date: e.g., medication errors reduction, doctor complaints)

Table 11.3. Low Cost/Best Value.

Tactical Plan Elements

Break down BHAG into quarterly work agendas

Reengineering and role changes in finance (Less "controls," more enabling of innovation and entrepreneurial activity)

Act on high-cost, high-volume processes

Maximize cash flow management

Management of private pay customer collection

Create bill customers can understand

Synchronize planning, budget, and operational cycles (often disconnected in many hospitals)

Power up staff down time (What tasks can be done during slow times?)

Cut approval levels and signatures

Incentivize cutting crap, forms, meetings

Set decision time standards on approvals

Outsource or discontinue side operations

Identify customer "waiting time" areas (opportunity for Length of Stay reduction and satisfaction)

Patient prep protocols associated with wait times

Rebid contracts annually (no long-term contracts)

Tie pay to personal and organizational performance

Purchasing standards and suppliers reduction

Work flow software

Physician economic credentialing

Economic value added (EVA) focus

Best-in-class tools—no cheap stuff, "deals"

Rapid information system integration of clinical, financial, support

Monthly and weekly tangibles/intangibles metrics (Set specific subgoals to reach by date: e.g., cost reductions, process hours saved)

Table 11.4. Best People/Best Team.

Tactical Plan Elements

Break down BHAG into quarterly work agendas

Move to values centered management asap

Revamp HR department and processes (Build cadre of people needed for business growth)

1st year training standard of 40 hours

Training for all:
　Values and cultural expectations
　Guest relations and team communication
　Ideation: problem solving and implementation

No pay increases without needed job training

Cost effective training
　Fewer outside courses
　JIT training

Aggressively reduce turnover to protect new people investments

Intellectual capital management review

Management development and muscle-building

Cross training/multi skilling for job flex

Redesign jobs per reengineering: no layoffs

Pay for performance; end non merit increases

Best only: tighten selection and promotion

Cultural redefinition, socialization, celebration

Worklife environment reengineering

Meet associate support needs (e.g., day care)

Correct or remove problem staff

Fewer levels/layers; consolidate departments

Fit the organization to what works for people

Monthly and quarterly outcomes metrics (Set specific subgoals to reach by date: e.g., morale scores, ideation rates, turnover)

Table 11.5. A Tactical Plan Format.

Customer Tactical Plan — 1st Quarter

A. Initiative Area: Irritations Removal

Identified Tasks	Assignee	Approach	$ Estimate	Target Date
1. Phone greeting and time-to-answer	T. Moran	DIG	0	2/1
2. Wait time E.R.— draft new process	G. Alvarez	DIG	Unknown	2/15
3. Patient billing and collections	J. Gonzalez	JDI	2000	3/1
4. ID admitting moments of truth	M. Jensen		0	1/15
5. Etc.				

B. Initiative Area: Physician Value Added Items

Identified Tasks	Assignee	Approach	$ Estimate	Target Date
1. DIG training for office staffs	K. Silber	DIG	1000	4/1
2. Communication re org transform	D. Hickey	JDI	0	1/22
3. Implement on-line lab results	M. Gosh	JDI	7000	2/7
4. Etc.				

C. Initiative Area: Service Improvements

Identified Tasks	Assignee	Approach	$ Estimate	Target Date
1. Patient shower in ER	J. Blowe	JDI	1000	3/15
2. Etc.				

of financing, desire to cluster related changes for greater impact, and so forth. Because there are four tactical plans (Customer, quality, cost, people), BHAG councils review and coordinate with each other to increase impact and avoid duplication. At the end of the year new tactical plans are drawn up for the following period, but the departure point in the second year of change is from the far higher altitude achieved in the first year.

What does all this produce? What is it reasonable to expect? Teams that can envision a new age of health care and then aggressively manage toward that dream will be rewarded at the end of the first year with an amazing change in the organization's ability to perform. BHAG's will have been met or at least approached. Better financial, clinical, Customer satisfaction, and human outcomes will be apparent and measurable. Success translates into larger market share, a shift in the job applicant traffic as the best people and physicians seek you out, and payer volumes that begin to shift in your direction. Doing the work, and then seeing the results, releases Associates' pride, a pride that people always feel when they know they've participated in creating something greater than themselves. These results are predictable, and the model of change that has been presented has proved reliable.

Standardize Islands, then Continents

Talking recently with my family physician I learned that his practice group wants to leave the paper patient folder era behind and adopt a computerized medical records program that he could use within his own office. As an "early adopter" of digital toys and tools, he reports that such programs are all over the map in terms of both content and format. A real problem for his practice is that it would benefit his group of seven physicians, but they might have to redo everything later on when the two hospitals he practices in make their individual decisions in terms of offering programs that will link to his office. What should he do?

I pointed out that with the installation of the new system in his office, an island of standardization would be created immediately among the seven physicians. The quality of record keeping would be improved immediately, drug interactions could be checked, and speed of access improved. He immediately would gain the benefit that this island would afford, and that is a lot better than standing in the swamp of the old paper system. Likewise, the hospitals would be creating their own, bigger islands of standardization, thus offering him a better place in which to practice.

The ideal would be if all best practices could first be identified and we could get there in one step, but that is not likely to happen. Effective management knows that islands can later be joined, in my physician's case either by a software translation program to convert to whatever the regional records format becomes, or, God forbid, by doing more hand entry. What results is first an island, then an archipelago, and then an emerging continent. When you're not sure about how to build a continent, make an island.

We're seeing a similar evolution in smart homes. Currently we have separate wires coming into the house for power, television, cable, and telephone. All kinds of subwiring is found inside the house for security systems, intercoms, and stereo. And then there are individual electrical appliances, outlets, and switches. The concept of the smart home is that these islands of invention will be connected and centrally controlled. So, too, will health care's best practices evolve closer to an integrated wholeness. It's going to be really neat to see it.

Raising standards in American health care to the level of best practices and beyond, and standardizing operations across the country to that level, is the mission to which we are called. The journey, like all those worth taking, is arduous, the way difficult. But it is a doable journey, and you are personally invited to make the trip. When those you lead see their organization crossing the goal line, when they stand in the winner's circle, the difficulties along the way will be forgotten. That is when one's fullest appreciation of what it means to be a pro's pro in management is realized.

Conclusion

This chapter has provided an organizing scheme, a sequence of change design, and suggestions for creating and successfully implementing tactical plans. As a concluding chapter it provides a beginning road map for next steps in what can be the most exciting journey of your career. We enter the new century with the knowledge that standardizing health care's best practices across the country is now possible, thereby delivering what our fellow citizens, and perhaps our own families, need and expect from us. Will this be difficult work? Yes, and it will demand the best that is in us. Would you want it any other way?

Work-Out Session

1. The first practical problem is deciding whether there is readiness for change among executives. Who among them wants to make change? Visit with them to discuss their ideas and views of the issues.
2. Would there be value in setting up a project team to study the feasibility of a standardization project in your organization? What existing initiatives might be drawn together to help achieve this?
3. Rather than chew up a lot of time debating the value of system standardization, or getting lost in the political ramifications or organizational questions, begin by drawing up a list of all the elements of the organization's performance people think need to be changed. Keep their "eyes on the prize" of what the organization could evolve into so as to shrink present concerns to their proper perspective.
4. What BHAGs would we like to achieve? Identify some grand goals; create long work lists to get there.
5. What pieces of work need fixing? What departments need improving?
6. Ask the group to commit. It's time to call the question.

Epilogue

According to ancient legend, Gordius, though a peasant, became King of Phrygia after being selected by the oracle at Delphi. To remind himself of his humble beginnings, he tied his peasant cart to a post in front of his palace with an enormous and intricate knot, and dedicated it to the deity. On his death, the people again journeyed to the oracle for a prophecy and were told that whoever unraveled the knot tied by Gordius would be their next ruler and the ruler of all Asia.

Years passed, and many tried unsuccessfully to untie the Gordian knot and claim rulership, but the knot remained fast. Eventually, the young Alexander, later called Great by the Romans, traveled to Phrygia flanked by a large army. The elders presented to him the problem and said they would submit to him if he could undo the knot. Hearing this, he drew his sword and cut through it with one stroke.

What will history say of us? What will historians write of health care leaders at the beginning of the twenty-first century? Perhaps they will write that although we had created dazzling life-saving science and medical breakthroughs, our health care organizations' very existence was threatened by a management approach hopelessly out of date and with bleak prospects for remaining viable. The contrast was stark: A promising health care future beckoned ahead, but with so many difficulties at the door, it seemed impossible to extricate the health care system from the sinkhole of outmoded management concepts.

I believe, however, that history will record that men and women of this generation provided the pivotal leadership that set organizational management on a new course. They intuitively understood that they had to look at the problem in new ways, and then got to work decisively to cut through it. Turning from old, unworkable, unwanted "solutions," they forged a brave new future, releasing the power of their people and building renewed and reborn systems of care. The American example became a standard to the world, and hundreds of millions of lives were blessed. America's benchmark health care delivery system was a beacon of hope. People were cured instead of merely treated, and the resources saved were deployed to repair society's other ills. These leaders made a difference. They were vital. It wouldn't have happened without them.

It won't happen without you.

References

Adelman, S. H. "A Proposed New Clearinghouse for Critical Pathways." www.msms.org/adelman/sa-8.htm. (n.d.)

Agency for Health Care Policy Research. "AHCPR, AAHP, and AMA to Develop National Clinical Guideline Clearinghouse." Press release, May 28, 1997.

Agency for Health Care Policy Research. "AHCPR Invites Clinical Practice Guidelines for Public/Private National Guideline Clearinghouse." Press release, April 13, 1998.

American College of Healthcare Executives (ACHE) 1996 publication.

American Heritage Dictionary of the English Language. Boston: Houghton-Mifflin, 1992.

American Productivity and Quality Center. http://www.apqc.org/. 1998.

American Society for Training and Development Benchmarking Forum. www.astd.org.

"America's Best Hospitals: Behind the Rankings." *U.S. News & World Report,* Aug. 12, 1996, p. 65.

Anderson, L. "Health Care Debate: 'Real Nurses vs. Unlicensed Aides." *Chicago Tribune,* Dec. 8, 1996, pp. 1, 17.

Balm, G. J. *Benchmarking: A Practitioner's Guide for Becoming and Staying Best of the Best.* Schaumburg, Ill.: Quality Productivity Management Association, 1992.

Bates, D. W., et al. "Incidence of Adverse Drug Events and Potential Adverse Drug Events." *Journal of the American Medical Association,* July 5, 1995, pp. 35–43.

"Beat the Budget and Astound Your CFO." *Fortune,* Oct. 28, 1996, pp. 187–189.

"Bedside ICU Computers Aid Direct Care." *Modern Healthcare,* Nov. 18, 1991, p. 26.

Bendell, T., Boulter, L., and Goodstadt, P. *Benchmarking for Competitive Advantage.* London: Pitman, 1997.

"The Big Payoff from Computers." *Fortune,* March 7, 1994, p. 28.

Blake, R., and Mouton, J. *The Managerial Grid.* Houston: Gulf, 1994. (Originally published 1964.)

Bogdanich, W. *The Great White Lie: How America's Hospitals Betray Our Trust and Endanger Our Lives.* New York: Simon & Schuster, 1991.

Brandon, K. "Doctor's Winning Suit Puts Managed Care on Trial." *Chicago Tribune,* April 26, 1998, sec. 1, p. 4.

Brennan, T., Leape, L., Laird, N., et al. "Incidence of Adverse Events and Negligence in Hospitalized Patients: Results of the Harvard Medical Practice Study I." *New England Journal of Medicine,* February 7, 1991, 370–376.

Burda, D. "JCAHO Still Pulling in Big Profits." *Modern Healthcare,* Nov. 28, 1994, p. 18.

Caggiano, C. "The Profit-Promoting Daily Scorecard." *Inc. Magazine,* May 1994, p. 101 ff.

Camp, R. C. *Benchmarking: The Search for Industry Best Practices that Lead to Superior Performance.* Milwaukee: SQC Quality Press, 1989.

Camp, R. C. *Business Process Benchmarking.* New York: Quality Resources, 1995.

Carollo, R., and Nesmith, J. www.austin360.com/news/features/milmed/milmed06.htm. 1977.

Case, J. "Games Companies Play." *Inc. Magazine,* Oct. 1994, p. 46 ff.

Center for Study of Services, 1994. *Consumer's Guide to Hospitals.* American Hospital Association.

"Chrysler Will Reduce Number of Suppliers," *Chicago Tribune,* 1995.

Codling, S. *Best Practice Benchmarking. The Management Guide.* London: Industrial Newsletters, 1992.

Codling, S. "If You Stop Getting Better You Stop Getting Good." www.metabpr.com/sylvia. (n.d.)

Colvin, G. "The Changing Art of Becoming Unbeatable." *Fortune,* Nov. 24, 1997, pp. 299–300.

"Competing Through Standardization." *Business Week,* Oct. 16, 1995.

The Concise Columbia Encyclopedia. New York: Columbia University Press, 1995.

"Counting What Counts." *Forbes ASAP,* April 7, 1997, p. 31 ff.

Dame, L., and Wolfe, S. "The Failure of 'Private' Hospital Regulation." *Public Citizen,* July 1996.

Deming, E. *Out of Crisis.* Cambridge, Mass.: MIT Press, 1986.

Drucker, P. "Management's New Paradigms." *Forbes,* Oct. 5, 1998, pp. 152–176.

"Drug Prescribing Errors Studied." *Modern Healthcare,* Jan. 27, 1997, p. 16.

Dunlap Godsey, K. "Slow Climb to New Heights: Combine Strict Discipline with Goofy Antics and Make Billions." *Success,* Oct. 1996, pp. 20–26.

Edmund, D. S. "The Secret Behind the Big Mac? It's Simple!" *Management Review,* May 1990, pp. 32–33.

Edvinsson, L., and Malone, M. *Intellectual Capital: Realizing Your Company's True Value by Finding Its Hidden Roots.* New York: Harper Business, 1997.

Emerson, R. W. "Self-Reliance." *Self-Reliance and Other Essays.* London: Dover, 1993. (Originally published in 1841.)

Fleishman, E. *Leadership Opinion Questionnaire.* New York: McGraw-Hill/ London House, 1989.

"For Good Outcomes, More Is Better." *Modern Healthcare,* Dec. 22–29, 1997, p. 44.

Fuchsberg, G. "Business Schools Get Bad Grades." *Wall Street Journal,* June 6, 1990.

Gardner, J. "VA Leads the Way." *Modern Healthcare,* Dec. 1, 1997.

Gardner, J. "Web Now Watchdog on Nursing Homes." *Modern Healthcare,* Oct. 26, 1998.

Grant, L. "Happy Workers, High Returns." *Fortune,* Jan. 12, 1998, p. 81.

Greene, J. "Florida 2nd State to Issue 'Report Cards.'" *Modern Healthcare,* March 4, 1996, p. 80.

Greer, O. L., et al. "The Key to Real Teamwork: Understanding the Numbers," *Management Accounting,* May 1992, p. 39 ff.

Grolier Encyclopedia. CD-ROM. Los Angeles: Philips Media Electronic Publishing, 1998.

Havighurst, C. Editorial. *Modern Healthcare,* Nov. 16, 1992.

Hayes, R. "Managing Our Way to Economic Decline." *Harvard Business Review,* July-Aug. 1980, pp. 67–77.

"HCIA Launches Hospital Database." *Modern Healthcare,* Feb. 23, 1998, p. 38.

HCIA-Mercer. "Implications of the Benchmark Study." HCIA's 100 Top Hospitals Studies for 1994, 1995, 1997. www.HCIA.com.

HCIA-Mercer. "100 Top Hospitals Studies, 1994–1998."

Health Information and Management Systems Society. "The Ninth Annual HIMSS Annual Leadership Survey." Feb. 1998. www.himss.org.

Helfrick, J. "Helping Hospitals Learn from Their Mistakes." *Modern Healthcare,* Jan. 18, 1999, p. 24.

Henkoff, R. "Growing Your Company: Five Ways to Do It Right." *Fortune,* Nov. 25, 1996, pp. 78–81.

Hensley, S. "The Deciding Vote." *Modern Healthcare,* Nov. 24, 1997, p. 42.

Hensley, S. "Pharmacists Get Rx." *Modern Healthcare,* Feb. 23, 1998a, p. 104.

Hensley, S. "Help from a Friend." *Modern Healthcare,* July 13, 1998b, p. 50.

"A Hero Without a Company." *Forbes,* March 18, 1991.

Herzlinger, R. E. *Market Driven Health Care.* Reading, Mass.: Addison-Wesley, 1997.

"How Market Leaders Keep Their Edge." *Fortune,* Feb. 6, 1995, p. 88 ff.

"IHF Congress Highlights." *Modern Healthcare International,* Nov., 1997, p. 14.

"Industry's Troubles Threaten to Trigger Leadership Paralysis." *Modern Healthcare,* Aug. 17, 1998, p. 28.

"In Light of Fraud Stories, Industry Should Focus on Reassuring Public." *Modern Healthcare,* July 28, 1997, p. 23.

"In Search of Evidence." *Modern Healthcare,* Nov. 9, 1998, p. 108.

"Invest in Companies that Invest in Workers." *Money,* March 1996.

"Is the Baldrige Overblown?" *Fortune,* July 1, 1991.

Jaklevic, M. C. "Providers Seek to Survey Satisfaction." *Modern Healthcare,* Aug. 5, 1995.

Jaklevic, M. C. "Marketers Gear Up for Quality Ratings." *Modern Healthcare,* April 1, 1996, p. 49.

Jaklevic, M. C. "Setting the Standard." *Modern Healthcare,* Sept. 7, 1998.

Jaklevic, M. C. "Hospital Report-Card Model in Peril." *Modern Healthcare,* Jan. 18, 1999, pp. 14–15.

"*JAMA:* 'Best Hospitals' List Just a Popularity Contest." *Modern Healthcare,* April 14, 1997. (The *JAMA* issue cited was April 8, 1997)

Japsen, B. "Survey: Money, Not Mission, Driving Mergers." *Modern Healthcare,* Oct. 13, 1997, p. 14.

Jones, T., and Sasser, E., Jr. "Why Satisfied Customers Defect." *Harvard Business Review,* Nov.-Dec. 1995, p. 88 ff.

Kaiser Permanente. *Annual Report,* 1994. Oakland, Calif.: Kaiser Permanente.

Kanter, R. M. "How to Compete." *Harvard Business Review,* March-April 1991.

Kaplan, R. S. *The Rise and Fall of Managerial Accounting.* Boston: Harvard Business School Press, 1991.

Kaplan, R. S., and Norton, D. P. "The Balanced Scorecard: Measures that Drive Performance." *Harvard Business Review,* Jan.-Feb. 1992, p. 71 ff.

Kaplan, R. S., and Norton, D. P. "Putting the Balanced Scorecard to Work." *Harvard Business Review,* Sept.-Oct. 1993, p. 134 ff.

Kaplan, R. S., and Norton, D. P. *The Balanced Scorecard: Translating Strategy into Action.* Boston: Harvard Business School Press, 1996.

Karlgaard, R. "SEC Loves IC." *Forbes ASAP,* April 7, 1997, p. 39 ff.

"Keeping It Simple: Airlines Standardize Fleets to Save Time, Cash." *Chicago Tribune,* Aug. 28, 1994.

Kertesz, L. "Horror Stories Aside, HMOs May Be Curbing Malpractice." *Modern Healthcare,* Aug. 5, 1996, pp. 56, 60.

Kertesz, L. "PacifiCare Does an Oxford." *Modern Healthcare,* Dec. 1, 1997, p. 4.

Kertesz, L. "Stays Still Too Long, Firm Says." *Modern Healthcare,* Jan. 19, 1998, pp. 20–21.

Klein, D. *Strategic Management of Intellectual Capital.* Portsmouth, N.H.: Heinemann, 1997.

Kurtzman, J. "Is Your Company Off Course? Now You Can Find Out Why." *Fortune,* Feb. 17, 1997, pp. 128–130.

Labich, K. "Is Herb Kelleher America's Best CEO?" *Fortune,* May 2, 1994, pp. 44–52.

Leape, L., Brennan, T., Laird, N., et al. "The Nature of Adverse Events in Hospitalized Patients: Results of the Harvard Medical Practice Study II." *New England Journal of Medicine,* Feb. 7, 1991, pp. 377–384.

"Lesson Still Isn't Getting Through: Bigger Isn't Better." *Modern Healthcare,* Nov. 18, 1996, p. 32.

Levering, R., and Moskowitz, M. *The 100 Best Companies to Work for in America.* New York: Plume, 1994.

Levering, R., and Moskowitz, M. "The 100 Best Companies to Work for in America." *Fortune,* Jan. 12, 1998, pp. 84–95.

Limbacher, P. B. "How Far Up Will It Go?" *Modern Healthcare,* Aug. 4, 1997, p. 2.

Linden, D. W., with Brennan, J., and Lane, R. "Another Boom Ends." *Forbes,* Jan. 20, 1992, pp. 76–80.

Love, J. F. *McDonald's: Behind the Arches.* New York: Bantam, 1995, pp. 119–126, 327–333. Copyright © 1986 by John F. Love. Used by permission of Bantam Books, a division of Random House, Inc.

Lowe, J. *Jack Welch Speaks: Wisdom from the World's Greatest Business Leader.* New York: Wiley, 1998.

Malone, M. "New Metrics for a New Age." *Forbes ASAP,* April 7, 1997, p. 40 ff.

Marriott, J. W., and Brown, K. A. The Spirit to Serve: Marriott's Way. San Francisco: HarperBusiness, 1997.

"Massachusetts to Publish Doc Profile Data." *Modern Healthcare,* Aug. 5, 1996, pp. 6, 8.

"A Master Class in Radical Change." *Fortune,* December 13, 1993, pp. 82–90.

McDonald's website: www.mcdonald's.com

McLaughlin, N. "Lookin' Bad: JCAHO-Hospital Fight a Disservice to Quality Healthcare." *Modern Healthcare,* Jan. 25, 1999, p. 24.

Memmott, M. "Productivity Gallops Past Expectations." *USA Today,* Aug. 9, 1995, p. B1.

Meyer, C. "How the Right Measures Help Teams Excel." *Harvard Business Review,* May-June 1994, p. 95 ff.

"Missouri Hospital Pleads No Contest to Fraud." *Modern Healthcare,* Sept. 2, 1996, p. 37.

Modern Healthcare, May 2, 1994.

Modern Healthcare, December 19, 1994, p. 2.

Moore, D. "A Higher Standard." *Modern Healthcare,* Oct. 26, 1998a, p. 14.

Moore, D. "Study Ties Staffing, Complications." *Modern Healthcare,* Dec. 7, 1998b, p. 3.

Moore, D. "A Slow Trickledown." *Modern Healthcare,* Sept. 14, 1998c, p. 70.

Moore, J. "Huge Savings Expected from New EDI Standards." *Modern Healthcare,* Sept. 9, 1996, pp. 18–19.

Moore, J. "Knowing the Score." *Modern Healthcare,* Nov. 23, 1998a, p. 38.

Moore, J. "Research Clearinghouse." *Modern Healthcare,* Aug. 24, 1998b.

Moore, J. "Testing the Waters." *Modern Healthcare,* June 1, 1998c, p. 26.

Moore, J. D., Jr. "Hospital Staff Cuts May Be Slowing." *Modern Healthcare,* Dec. 16, 1996, pp. 28–30.

Moore, J. D., Jr. "SEIU Takes Aim." *Modern Healthcare,* Jan. 27, 1997a, p. 8.

Moore, J. D., Jr. "Labor Gets Tough." *Modern Healthcare,* March 10, 1997b, p. 32.

Moore, J. D., Jr. "An SEIU Victory." *Modern Healthcare,* Nov. 3, 1997c, p. 30.

Morrissey, J. "Delayed Breast Cancer Diagnosis Leading Cause of Lawsuits—Study." *Modern Healthcare,* June 5, 1995.

Morrissey, J. "HEDIS to Expand Performance Guidelines," *Modern Healthcare,* July 22, 1996a, pp. 2–3.

Morrissey, J. "Performance Comparisons Gaining." *Modern Healthcare,* Jan. 15, 1996b, p. 33.

Morrissey, J. "Alliance Prepares to Roll Out Proposed Performance Measures." *Modern Healthcare,* March 25, 1996c, p. 54.

Morrissey, J. "Stalled on the On-Ramp." *Modern Healthcare,* March 10, 1997a.

Morrissey, J. "Columbia Info System Strategy in Question Under Restructuring." *Modern Healthcare,* Dec. 1, 1997b, p. 4.

Morrissey, J. "Who Needs Paper?" *Modern Healthcare,* Sept. 1, 1997c, p. 72.

Morrissey, J. "Integrated in Name Only." *Modern Healthcare,* Jan. 5, 1998a, p. 36.

Morrissey, J. "Information Systems Evangelists." *Modern Healthcare,* Feb. 23, 1998b, pp. 70–84.

Morrissey, J. "Massachusetts Group Targets Medical Mistakes." *Modern Healthcare,* Aug. 17, 1998c, p. 16.

Morrissey, J. "All Benchmarked Out." *Modern Healthcare,* Dec. 7, 1998d, pp. 38–46.

National Health Care Skill Standards Project. Benefits listed on Internet site. www.fwl.org/nhcssp/health.

"New HEDIS Measures Give Providers Chance to Mature." *Modern Healthcare,* July 22, 1996, p. 26.

O'Reilly, B. "Reengineering the MBA." *Fortune,* Jan. 24, 1994, p. 38 ff.

Otter, J. P. "Leading Change: Why Transformation Efforts Fail." *Harvard Business Review,* March-April, 1995, pp. 59–67.

Pagonis, W. G. "The Work of a Leader." *Harvard Business Review,* Nov.-Dec. 1992, pp. 118–126.

Pallarito, K. "More Hospitals Settle." *Modern Healthcare,* Sept. 8, 1997, p. 36.

Peters, T. "Service or Perish." *Forbes ASAP,* Dec. 4, 1995, p. 144.

Peters, T., and Waterman, R. *In Search of Excellence.* New York: G. K. Hall, 1984, 1997.

Porter, M. E. *Competitive Strategy: Techniques for Analyzing Industries and Competitors.* New York: Free Press, 1998a.

Porter, M. E. *Competitive Advantage: Creating and Sustaining Superior Performance.* New York: Free Press, 1998b.

"Quality of Care Declining, SEIU Survey Says." *Modern Healthcare,* Dec. 22–29, 1998, p. 16.

"Rate Your Readiness to Change." *Fortune,* Feb. 7, 1994.

Reichheld, F. "Learning from Customer Defections." *Harvard Business Review,* March-April 1996, p. 56 ff.

Roberts, J., Coale, J., and Redman, R. "A History of the Joint Commission on Accreditation of Hospitals." *Journal of the American Medical Association,* Aug. 21, 1987, p. 938.

Schaffer, R. H., and Thomson, H. A. "Successful Change Programs Begin with Results." *Harvard Business Review,* Jan.-Feb. 1992, pp. 80–89.

Schlesinger, L. A., and Heskett, J. L. "The Service-Driven Service Company." *Harvard Business Review,* Sept.-Oct. 1991, pp. 71–81, 146–158.

Schonfeld, E. "Can Computers Cure Health Care?" *Fortune,* March 10, 1998, internet edition at www.pathfinder.com/fortune/1998/980330/hea.html.

Scott, L. "Limiting Waste in the Supply Chain." *Modern Healthcare,* April 22, 1996, p. 48.

Scott, L. "Not Together Yet." *Modern Healthcare,* Jan. 5, 1997, p. 36.

Sherman, S. *Growing People for Peak Performance.* San Francisco: Jossey-Bass. Forthcoming.

Sherman, V. C. "Unionism and the Nonunion Company." *Personnel Journal,* June 1969, pp. 413–422.

Sherman, V. C. "What Exactly Do Aides Do?" *Inservice Training and Education,* Nov. 1974.

Sherman, V. C. *From Losers to Winners: How to Manage Problem Employees and What to Do If You Can't.* New York: American Management Association, 1987.

Sherman, V. C. *Creating the New American Hospital: A Time for Greatness.* San Francisco: Jossey-Bass, 1993.

Sherman, V. C. "Organization Performance and Readiness Assessment." Available at www.managementhouse.com.

Shinkman, R. "Industry Taking New Look at Medical Error Casualties." *Modern Healthcare,* Oct. 21, 1996a, p. 12.

Shinkman, R. "Two Medpartners Execs out of Jobs, Facing Lawsuits." *Modern Healthcare,* Dec. 2, 1996b, p. 8.

"Sixty Percent of Facilities Cut Staffing—Study." *Modern Healthcare,* March 10, 1997, p. 32.

Skinner, W. "The Focused Factory." *Harvard Business Review,* May-June 1974; cited in Herzlinger, 1997.

"Slow Climb to New Heights: Combine Strict Discipline with Goofy Antics and Make Billions." *Success,* Oct. 1996, pp. 20–26.

Snow, C. "Apria to Pay $1.7 Million to Settle Kickback Charges." *Modern Healthcare,* Dec. 16, 1996, p. 16.

Stack, J. "Mad About Layoffs." *Inc. Magazine,* May 1996, pp. 21–22.

Stewart, T. "Your Company's Most Valuable Asset: Intellectual Capital." *Fortune,* Oct. 3, 1994.

Stewart, T. A. *Intellectual Capital: The New Wealth of Organizations.* New York: Doubleday, 1997.

Strathern, P. *Hegel in 90 Minutes.* Chicago: Ivan R. Dee, 1997.

"System Follows Protocol to Fight Disease." *Modern Healthcare,* Oct. 26, 1998, p. 56.

"Tale of Health Care Could Induce Nausea." *USA Today,* Dec. 15, 1991.

Taylor, C. *Hegel and Modern Society.* Cambridge: Cambridge University Press, 1979.

Teal, T. "The Human Side of Management." *Harvard Business Review,* Nov.-Dec. 1996, pp. 35–44.

Thurow, L. "Where Management Fails." *Newsweek,* Dec. 7, 1981, p. 78.

Top-ix Ltd. "Business Process Benchmarking." www.metabr.com/benchmark.

Treacy, M., and Wiersmas, F. *The Discipline of Market Leaders: Choose Your Customers, Narrow Your Focus, Dominate Your Market.* Menlo Park, Calif.: Addison-Wesley, 1997.

"Two Hospitals Latest to Settle Patient 'Dumping' Cases." *Modern Healthcare,* Oct. 7, 1996, p. 44.

Walton, S., with Huey, J. *Sam Walton: Made in America.* New York: Doubleday, 1992, pp. 246–249.

Watson, G. H. *The Benchmarking Workbook.* Portland, Ore.: Productivity Press, 1992.

Weidner, C. K. "Southwest Airlines." Chicago: Management House, Inc., 1990.

Weissenstein, E., and Moore, D. "Quality Under Scrutiny." *Modern Healthcare,* Sept. 28, 1998, p. 12.

Welch, J. "GE Letter to Shareholders." Feb. 7, 1997.

"What Flexible Workers Can Do." *Fortune,* Feb. 1989.

Winslow, R. "Computers Helping Doctors Match Care with Costs Can Lower Bills, Study Says." *Wall Street Journal,* June 20, 1993, p. B6.

Woodyard, C. "Columbia/HCA Lawsuits Plague Stock Holding." *USA Today,* Aug. 20, 1997, p. B3.

Zairi, M. *Competitive Benchmarking: An Executive Guide.* Houston: Gulf Publishing.

Appendix A: MANSYS Management System

Table of Contents

IV. Manage Work
   A. Time Managing for Results
      1. The Key Results Hour
      2. Meeting Management
      3. Other Time Tips
      4. Basic Tools: Calendar, Contacts, and To Do
   B. Planned Performance: Work Planning and Specification
   C. Planned Performance: Review and Development
   D. Work Gating
   E. Making Delegation Work
   F. Priority Evaluation and Protection
   G. Improve Work Processes

V. Drive Change
   A. Change Managing
      1. Creative Destruction
      2. Getting Ideas and Gathering Knowledge
      3. Innovation Management and Intellectual Capital
   B. Fast Action With Teams and Individuals
   C. Proposal Selling
      What Executives Want in a Proposal
   D. Conflict Management
      1. Personal Conflict Management
      2. Organization Conflict Management

Appendix B: Web Sites Related to Standardization

Many of these sites have links or are useful departure points. All web addresses were checked before publication but may have been changed.

Search Engines

http://altavista.digital.com/	AltaVista
http://www.amazon.com/	Amazon Books
http://ultra.infoseek.com/	Infoseek
http://www.yahoo.com/	Yahoo!

Quality Sites

http://www.apqc.org/	American Productivity and Quality Center
http://www.asqc.org/	American Society for Quality Control
http://web5.whs.osd.mil/	Defense Department Office of Quality Management
http://www.nahq.org/	National Association for Health Care Quality
http://www.fwl.org/nhcssp/	National Health Care Skill Standards Project
http://www.guideline.gov/	National Guidelines Clearinghouse

Associations and Agencies

http://www.ahcpr.gov/	Agency for Health Care Policy and Research

http://207.96.21.130/	American Association of Integrated Health Care Delivery Systems
http://www.ama-assn.org	American Medical Association
http://amia2.amia.org/	American Medical Informatics Association
http://www.astd.org/	American Society for Training and Development
http://www.cdc.gov/nchswww/	Centers for Disease Control
http://www.fahs.com/	Federation of American Health Systems
http://www.hanys.org/resource/links/	Health Association of New York (great links)
http://www.himss.org/	Health Care Information and Management Systems Society
http://www.nahc.org/	National Association for Home Care
http://www.podi.com/nbch/	National Business Coalition on Health
http://www.nih.gov/	National Institutes of Health

Publishers/Consultants

http://www.amhpi.com/default.htm	American Hospital Publishing
http://www1.mosby.com/	Best Practices and Benchmarking in Health Care
http://www.statpath.com/	Center for Health Education
http://www.iplabs.com/hr/	Human Resources Learning Center
http://www.ihs.on.ca/regulatory/health.htm	IHS Health Information
http://www.nursingcenter.com/	Lippincott's Nursing Center
http://www.managementhouse.com/	Management House (author's site)

http://www.modernhealthcare.com/	Modern Healthcare
http://www.benchnet.com/	The Benchmarking Exchange
http://www.benchmarking.co.uk/	The Benchmarking Center
http://www.vh.org/	Virtual Hospital

Standards Organizations

http://web.ansi.org/	American National Standards Institute
http://www.hcia.com/	HCIA Top 100 List
http://www.iso.ch/	International Organization for Standardization
http://www.jcaho.org/	Joint Commission on Accreditation of Healthcare Organizations
http://www.ncqa.org/	National Committee for Quality Assurance
http://www.quality.nist.gov/	National Institute of Standards and Technology (Baldrige Award)

Intellectual Capital and Knowledge Management

http://kman.bus.utexas.edu/kman/	Knowledge Management— University of Texas
http://www.knowledge.org.uk/	Knowledge On-Line
http://www.brint.com/km	WWW Virtual Library on Knowledge Management

Index

180. *See also* Automation; Computerization; Technology

Initiatives, strategic, listing, in balanced scorecard, 55–56

Injuries in hospitals, 6–7, 9, 91–92

Innovation capital, 182

Institute for Healthcare Quality, 164

Institute of Management Accountants, 46

Institute of Medicine, 198–199

Intangible measure, 172–176

Integrated information systems, 188–189

Integration: horizontal, 262; level of, in health care systems, 253–254; of physicians, 76; strategy of, 36–37; vertical, 255, 262. *See also* Consolidations; Health care systems

Intel, 156

Intellectual capital (IC): Associates as source of, 176, 177–178, 181, 206–207; automation and, 190–191; competitive advantage of, 168, 170, 175–176; computerization and, 184–190; currency of, 169–176; Customers as source of, 178–180, 182, 244; defined, 169–170; elements of, 180–182; estimating the value of, 172–176; examples of valuable, 172; financial measures and, 173–175; following indicators of, 170; human capital component of, 176, 177–178, 181; knowledge management of, 171, 176–182; leading indicators of, 170; locating, with organization, 176–177; measurement of, 177, 182–184; need for organizational learning and, 170–171; packaging, 179–180; Skandia approach to, 180–182; steps for using, 220–222; structural capital component of, 176, 178–179, 181–182; web sites about, 307. *See also* Associates; Health care; Ideas; Staff; Structural capital

Intellectual capital (IC) report, 182–183

Intellectual property, 182

Intermountain Health Care, 188–189

Internal bureaucratic load, 10

Internal competition, 109

Internal standards, 103–109; Customers as source of, 104–106; physicians as source of, 106–108; staff Associates as source of, 108–109. *See also* Best practices; Standards

Internet/World Wide Web: association and agency sites on, 305–306; best practices dissemination on, 189, 221–222, 234–235, 241; best practices sources on, 237–238, 305–307; for connectivity, 185–186; intellectual capital and knowledge management sites on, 307; for packaging intellectual capital, 179; physician credentials data on, 203; publisher and consultant sites on, 306–307; quality-related sites on, 305; search engines for, 305; searching, 238; security and confidentiality concerns about, 186, 190; standards organizations on, 307; usage of, by health care industry, 185–186

Intranets, 179, 190

J

J. D. Powers, 121

Jackson Hole Group, 121

Jaklevic, M. C., 112, 115, 118, 203

Japsen, B., 14

Job insecurity, 194

Job redesign, 208

Johnson & Johnson, 156

Johnson, K., 68

Joint Commission on Accreditation of Healthcare Organizations (JCAHO), 7; board representatives of, 94–95; changes at, 98–99; hospitals versus patients